NATIONAL AWARD WINNER

GALA

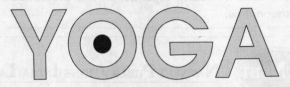

YOGASANA AND PRANAYAMA FOR HEALTH

by

Dr. P. D. Sharma

B. Sc., M. A., Ph. D., M. P. E., D. B. Ed.,
D. F. C. (Germany)

Translated by

Prof. R. M. Shah

M. A. LL. B.

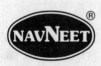

NAVNEET PUBLICATIONS (INDIA) LIMITED

Navneet House	**Navneet Bhavan**
Gurukul Road, Memnagar,	Bhavanishankar Road,
Ahmadabad – 380 052.	Dadar, Mumbai – 400 028.
(Tel. 2743 6300/2743 9300)	Phone : 5663 65

DHANLAL

70, Prince

S 202

G 505

Visit us at : www.navn

e-mail : npil@navneet.com   **Price : Rs. 30.00**

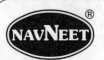 **NAVNEET PUBLICATIONS (INDIA) LIMITED**

Mumbai : 1. Bhavani Shankar Road, Dadar (West), **Mumbai – 400 028.** (Tel. 5662 6565 • Fax : 5662 6470)

2. **Navyug Distributors :** Road No. 8, M. I. D. C., Next to Indian Institute of Packaging, Marol, Andheri (East), **Mumbai – 400 093.** (Tel. 2821 4186 • Fax : 2835 2758)

Ahmadabad : Navneet House, Gurukul Road, Memnagar, **Ahmadabad – 380 052.** (Tel. 2743 6300/2743 9300)

Bangalore : No. 98, 1st Floor, 6th Cross, 6th Main, Malleswaram, **Bangalore – 560 003.** (Tel. 346 5740)

Bhopal : Navneet Sadan, E-7/728, Arera Colony, Shahpura, **Bhopal – 462 016.** (Tel. 527 8544)

Chennai : 30, Shriram Nagar, North Street, Alwarpet, **Chennai – 600 018.** (Tel. 2434 6404)

Delhi : 2E/23, Orion Plaza, 2nd & 3rd Floor, Jhandewalan Extn., **New Delhi – 110 055.** (Tel. 2361 0170)

Hyderabad : Bldg. No. 3-2-331, 2nd Floor, Somasundaram Street, **Secunderabad – 500 025.** (Tel. 5531 7348)

Kolkata : Newar Bhavan, 1st Floor, No. 87, Chowringhee Road, **Kolkata – 700 020.** (Tel. 2223 2497)

Nagpur : Agge Apartments, Agyaramdevi – S. T. Stand Road, **Nagpur – 440 018.** (Tel. 272 4411)

Patna : 1st Floor, 36-D, Sahdeo Mahto Marg, Srikrishnapuri, **Patna – 800 001.** (Tel. 20 4921)

Pune : Sita Park, 18, Shivaji Nagar, Near Bharat English School, **Pune – 411 005.** (Tel. 2553 6364)

Surat : 1, Ground Floor, Shree Vallabh Complex, Kotwal Street, Nanpara, **Surat – 395 001.** (Tel. 346 3927)

Vadodara : F/1, Vaidya Vatika, Opp. Hanuman Wadi, Sardar Bhuvan Khancho, **Vadodara – 390 001.** (Tel. 242 2087)

Dedication

Dedicated to my revered parents

– Dr. P. D. Sharma

PREFACE

Yoga as a system of physical exercise has been in existence in India since very ancient times. According to our ancient sages, there are eight stages of Yoga, namely Yama (Social Discipline), Niyama (Individual Discipline), Asana (Postures), Pranayama (Breath Control), Pratyahara (Mental Discipline), Dharana (Concentration), Dhyana (Meditation) and Samadhi (Self-realization). If an aspirant, after observing the disciplines of Yama and Niyama, practises Yogic exercises, his tubular channels are cleansed, he achieves excellent health and his mind becomes alert. This enables him to experience mental ecstasy. This book has been written for the common man. A humble effort has been made here to show through simple language and neat figures the usefulness and importance of Yogasana and Pranayama.

In this book, sixty-five important asanas have been explained and illustrated. Nowadays, Yoga is also used for the cure of several physical and mental ailments, and keeping this in view effects of Yogasana on more than forty diseases have been discussed. The asanas given in this book have been discussed from the point of view of their therapeutic use. So, the reader is not required to refer to any other books on the subject.

Along with Yogasanas, this book contains an explanation of the process of **Surya Namaskara.** Surya Namaskara is a complete exercise. The twelve stages of Surya Namaskara have been fully explained with figures with a view to enabling an aspirant to practise Surya Namaskara easily for maintaining his health. Besides this, their benefits have also been mentioned.

The practice of Yogasanas is incomplete without Pranayama. Hence a general explanation of **Pranayama** has been given with reference to health and Yogasanas.

To increase the utility of the book four new chapters **'The Purification of the Body Shatkarma Through Yoga'**, **'Yogasana and Exercises for the Care of the Eyes'**, **'A Suitable Diet'** and **'Model Yogasana-Timings'** have been added.

The book has been recommended to higher secondary schools, colleges and public libraries by the Curator of Libraries, Gujarat State, Gandhinagar, vide Circular Number 8224-8600 dated 8–10–1984.

This book received the **National Award** from the **Sports Authority of India** in the **XVII National Sports and Physical Education Books Competition.**

I am very thankful to Dr. Dhiren Gala for his valuable suggestions to make this book useful to persons belonging to all walks of life.

I am deeply obliged to Prof. R. M. Shah for this English version of my Gujarati book ''યોગાસન – પ્રાણાયામ કરો અને નીરોગી રહો''.

I am also grateful to M/s Gala Publishers for agreeing to publish this book.

—Dr. P. D. SHARMA

Principal, Sheth C. N. Vyayam Vidyabhavan,
Ambawadi, Ahmadabad–380 006.

SPORTS AUTHORITY OF INDIA

LAKSHMIBAI NATIONAL COLLEGE OF PHYSICAL EDUCATION, GWALIOR

Certificate of Honour

This Certificate of Honour is awarded to Shri ___Dr. P.D. Sharma___

___ for having received ___ Rs. 2,500/-

Prize in category ___SECOND___ in the 17th/18th National Prize Competition for Published Literature on Physical Education, Sports, Health Education, Recreation and Yoga at a function held at LNCPE, Gwalior, on 19th June, 1989

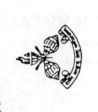

(Dr. A. K. UPPAL)
Prof. & Dean
L. N. C. P. E., Gwalior

(D. K. CHATTERJEE)
Director General
Sports Authority of India

CONTENTS

1. INTRODUCTION TO YOGA

Man has made tremendous progress in almost every walk of life. Objects once considered impossible to be achieved have now been achieved by us. What we have achieved and accomplished today could not have been imagined in their dreams by our past generations. Modern scientists and researchers have absolutely changed our life-style. Science has been incessantly pouring on us new materials and devices to make our physical life more happy and comfortable.

However, pollution of air, water, body and mind is also the result of science. We witness despair and disappointment on the faces of our young generation. Signs of restlessness are apparently visible in the dry and dull eyes of our young men and women. Sloping shoulders, flat chests and bulging stomachs have become their characteristics. Why?

Today, we can claim that we are modern and civilized but cannot claim that we are genuinely happy. We, today, use tranquillizers for sleep, pills for purgative and tonics for vigour. Tranquillizers and sedatives are in vogue in our modern society. Charmed by and then, addicted to intoxicative drugs, our youth is led to the path of disgrace and self-destruction.

Longing for material wealth has hardened our heart. Human values are declining. Work to time, competition and commotion have made us suffer from stress and strain. Mental tension or strain produces undesirable consequences. Stress and strain are the causes of physical as well as psychological diseases such as diabetes, cancer, acidity, ulcer, migraine and hypertension.

How can we prevent ourselves from being strained and degenerated? Should we discard science and scientific inventions? Should we return to the cave-life and live as the aborigines lived?

As a matter of fact, to do this is neither practical nor necessary. Yoga has the surest remedies for man's physical as well as psychological ailments. Yoga makes the organs of the body active in their functioning and has good effect on internal functioning of the human body. Yoga changes for good man's views on, and attitude to, life.

The word *yoga* is derived from the Sanskrit root *yuj* (युज्) meaning to bind the yoke. It is the true union of our will with the will of God.

Our ancient sages have suggested eight stages of Yoga to secure purity of body, mind and soul and final communion with God. These eight stages are known as **Ashtangayoga**. The eight stages of Yoga are as follows :

1. *Yama* (Social Discipline) : Yama means restraint or abstention. It contains five moral practices. They are :

Non-violence (*Ahimsa*), Truthfulness (*Satya*), Non-stealing (*Asteya*), Celibacy (*Brahmacharya*) and Non-acquisitiveness (*Aparigraha*).

Non-violence (*Ahimsa*) means not to hurt any creature mentally or physically through mind, speech or action. Truthfulness *(Satya) is the presentation of a matter as perceived with the help of sense organs. Non-stealing (Asteya)* means not to covet and acquire physically, mentally or by speech others' possessions.

Celibacy – Moderation in sex (*Brahmacharya*) : Brahmacharya does not mean lifelong celibacy, but moderation in sex between married couples.

Non-acquisitiveness (*Aparigraha)* means abandoning wealth and means of sensual pleasures.

2. *Niyama* (Individual Discipline) : Rules of conduct towards oneself consist of certain disciplines which are both physical and mental. These are five in number :

Cleanliness (*Shaucha*), Contentment (*Santosha*), Austerity (*Tapas*), Self-study (*Svadhyaya*) and Surrender to God (*Ishvara Pranidhana*).

Cleanliness (*Shaucha*) means internal and external purification of the body and the mind.

Contentment (*Santosha*) is a state of mind by which one

lives happily and satisfied in congenial or uncongenial atmosphere.

Austerity or penance (*Tapas*) is the conquest of all desires or sensual pleasures by practising purity in thought, speech and action.

Self-study (*Svadhyaya*) means exchange of thoughts in order to secure purity in thought and accomplish knowledge.

Surrender to God *(Ishvara Pranidhana)* : It consists of pure devotion to God and surrender of all actions to Him.

3. *Asana* (Postures) : Asana means holding the body in a particular posture to bring stability to the body and poise to the mind. The practice of asana brings purity in tubular channels, firmness to the body and vitality to the body and the mind. There are many asanas, but keeping in view a common man's health, 65 asanas have been presented and explained in this book.

4. *Pranayama* (Breath Control) : The literal meaning of Pranayama is **Breath Control.** The aim of practising Pranayama is to stimulate, regulate and harmonize vital energy of the body. Just as a bath is required for purifying the body, so also Pranayama is required for purifying the mind.

5. *Pratyahara* (Discipline of the Senses) : The extro-version of the sense organs due to their hankering after worldly objects has to be restrained and directed inwards towards the source of all existence. This process of drawing the sense inwards is Pratyahara or putting the sense under restraint.

6. *Dharana* (Concentration) : Dharana (Concentration) means focusing the pure mind on one's personal deity or on the Individual Self. The practice of Dharana helps the mind to concentrate on a particular object.

7. *Dhyana* (Meditation) : When one sustains and maintains the focus of attention through Dharana unbound by time and space, it becomes Dhyana (Meditation). Deep concentration destroys the Rajas and Tamas Gunas of mind and develops the Satvika Gunas (qualities).

8. *Samadhi* **(Self-realisation) :** The eighth and final stage of Yoga is Samadhi. At this stage, one's identity becomes both externally and internally immersed in meditation. The meditator, the act of meditation and the object meditated upon, all the three shed their individual characteristics and merge with one single vision of the entire cosmos. Supreme happiness, free from pleasure, pain or misery, is experienced. Samadhi is the climax of Dhyana.

The group of Dharana, Dhyana and Samadhi is called 'Samyama' (the Internal Yoga) in the Science of Yoga. The first five stages – Yama, Niyama, Asana, Pranayama and Pratyahara – constitute the External Yoga. If all these five stages are practised and followed in life, virtues like morality, morally sound conduct and good character are developed in man. Besides, there is all-round progress in human life, physically, intellectually and spiritually and man attains physical fitness and mental equanimity.

Thus, asanas are only one of the stages of Yoga. Most of the aspirants practising Yoga practise, in fact, these asanas. However, all the eight stages of Yoga are of importance. The practice of all the stages together and Pranayama bring a good deal of permanent benefits.

2. YOGASANAS *(The Yogic Postures)* : Importance, Rules and Classification

Yogasanas are simple actions for keeping the internal and external parts of the body in good health. No activity can be performed well so long as the internal and external parts of the body are not in good health. The body and the mind are closely interrelated. Both should be fully taken care of. Thousands of years ago, the people of ancient Greece believed in the principle 'A sound mind in a sound body'. The whole system of their education was based on this principle.

There are seven ways for the elimination of waste matter produced in the body by daily physical activities and functioning of the digestive system : (1) through left and right nostrils, (2) through left and right eyes, (3) through left and right ears, (4) through the mouth, (5) through the anus, (6) through the genitals and (7) through the skin. Most diseases are the result of the absence of sufficient and regular elimination of waste matter such as urine and stool from the body. Yogic exercises help the process of elimination of waste matter from the body and keep the body in perfectly sound health.

Importance : The reasons why Yogasanas have a preference over other systems of physical exercises are enumerated below :

(1) In other systems of physical exercise, the internal organs of the body do not get proper exercise, while Yogasanas give sufficient exercise to the internal organs of the body. Consequently, an individual can maintain good health and longevity of life.

(2) Only a small airy place and few equipments are required for practising Yogasanas.

(3) Two or more individuals are required in other games, while Yoga is a solo-practice.

(4) Yogasanas have a greater impact on the mind and the senses than other physical exercises with the result that

13

Yogasanas help to develop one's physical and mental powers to calm the mind and control the senses.

(5) The practice of Yogasanas is not expensive as one practising Yogasanas needs no additional food.

(6) There is sufficient elimination of stool and other waste matter from the body through Yogasanas and hence the body has more resistance power to keep a disease away.

(7) The body becomes flexible by Yogasanas. It becomes active with an increased ability of doing any activity. One who performs Yogasanas looks younger in age and lives longer.

(8) The blood in the different blood vessels is purified through different Yogasanas.

(9) The power of contraction and expansion of lungs is increased by practising Yogasanas and Pranayama. This results in the purification of blood to a great extent.

(10) Life span, youth and health depend upon the flexibility of the spinal cord. Yogasanas keep the spinal cord flexible.

(11) Asanas require the least possible use of physical energy. As a result, one feels less tired. This is the reason why Yogasanas are called a 'non-violent activity'.

(12) One who practises Yogasanas becomes a morally good person.

(13) Yogasanas help the mind to experience tranquillity. There is progressive intellectual development because of the calm mind.

(14) Yogasanas stimulate different glands of the body. These stimulated glands produce secretions in proper proportion, which having mixed with blood helps the body to acquire a well-balanced growth.

(15) Diseases like constipation, gas-trouble, diabetes, blood pressure, hernia, headache, etc. can be cured by practising Yogasanas and Pranayama.

(16) Yogasanas make possible not only physical and mental development but also intellectual and spiritual development.

(17) There is no restriction of age and sex for Yogasana aspirants. Our ancient sages had adopted this system for thousands of years with the result that they enjoyed sound health for a long time.

Hints : To take the full advantage of Yogasanas, it is advisable to follow the following points :

(1) For practising Yogasanas, early morning is the ideal time. Before starting Yoga practices, the bowels and the bladder should be emptied. It is better to do Yogasanas after a bath because it makes the body light and active and one can practise Yogasanas with greater ease. If one wishes to take a bath again after practising Yogasanas, one should use warm water instead of cold water.

(2) The ground for practising asanas should be level, clean and free from noise. Asanas should be practised on a mat or a carpet.

(3) Clothing should be in accordance with the season. Men should wear a loincloth or shorts. Women should wear a loose blouse and stretch pants.

(4) One should remain silent while practising asanas. While practising asanas, concentration should be on breathing and on the limbs which have a stress or strain. Concentration in the practice of Yogasanas is necessary for the all-round progress of the body and the mind.

(5) Before one begins to practise other asanas, one should perform Shavasana in order to make breathing normal, the body and the mind tranquil.

(6) Yogasana is a non-violent activity and therefore no force or jerk should be exerted in the practice of Yogasanas.

(7) There should be a gradual increase in the time duration in the practice of Yogasanas. By this process, the body becomes flexible and in a short time, it will easily accomplish a perfect state in each asana.

(8) Yogasana is a scientific process which deals with the internal and external parts of the body. A beginner should start practising Yogasanas after having learnt all their techniques under proper guidance.

(9) The performer of asanas should take light food in order to keep the body light.

(10) If one is suffering from complicated diseases or severe fever, one should not practise asanas. Women should not practise asanas four months after conception, for three months after delivery and during menstruation. A woman-aspirant should not as far as possible perform, without proper guidance asanas which involve lifting up the weight of the whole body on her hands.

(11) The number of asanas and the duration for each of them should be increased gradually. Practising many asanas on the first day should be avoided.

(12) Haste or quickness in coming to the final position from the initial position and *vice versa* should be avoided.

(13) After practising Yogasanas, Shavasana should be performed. Shavasana is a perfect asana. By Shavasana, the body gets speedy relaxation and becomes energetic.

(14) Yogasanas are supposed to be performed advantageously in the right direction if the aspirant, after practising Yogasanas, feels no tiredness and has an increased capacity to work with his light and refreshed body.

Classification of Yogasanas : In order to understand Yogasanas and study them well, they have been classified as follows in this book :

(1) Sitting Postures
(2) Supine Postures
(3) Abdominal Postures
(4) Hand-Postures
(5) Knee-Postures (Kneeling Postures)
(6) Leg-Postures (Standing Postures)
(7) Head-Postures

3. THE PURIFICATION OF THE BODY SHATKARMA THROUGH YOGA

Prior to practising Yogasana, Pranayama and meditation, it is desirable and also necessary to detoxify and purify the body. Toxic properties accumulate in the body for a number of reasons. If these toxins are not eliminated from the body, one would not get the desired benefits of Yogasanas and Pranayama.

The Yogashastra has shown six types of techniques (The kriyas) of internal purification. They are known as : neti, dhauti, nauli, basti, tratak and kapalbhati. A simple and brief information regarding the technique of purification has been given below :

(1) **Neti :** There are various methods of doing 'neti'. Here, only jalneti has been described.

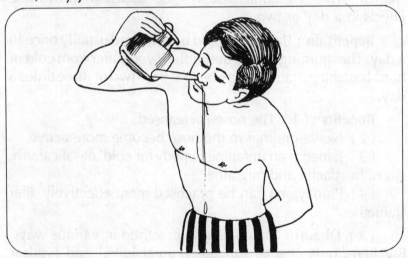

Neti

For doing 'Jalneti', a special kind of Jug–'netilota'–is used. Fill the jug with pure water. Add half a spoon of salt to it. First boil the water and then cool it. Stand in front of a basin or in a mori. Lower the head to the left side. Place the funnel of the jug into the right nostril. Further, lower the head slightly and raise the jug so that the water which entered the right nostril comes through the left nostril. Continue this 'kriya' for a minute. Then take the funnel out of the right nostril.

Now place the funnel of the jug into the left nostril and lower the head to the right side so that the water which entered the left nostril may come out of the right nostril. Continue this 'kriya' for a minute.

Then sneeze fifteen to twenty times (breathing out forcefully from the nose) and let the water be evacuated from the nose. It is necessary to make the nose dry.

Note : (1) If the water comes into the mouth through the nostril, spit it, do not swallow it.

(2) There will be burning sensation in the nose and, with frequent sneezes, the eyes will fill with tears while doing 'jalneti'. This is natural. You will be accustomed to these effects in a day or two.

Repetition : 'Jalneti' should be practised usually once in a day. The morning time is desirable. If you suffer from cold or hard-breathing, 'jalneti' may be practised two or three times a day.

Benefits : (1) The nose is cleansed.

(2) Nerve-endings in the nose become more active.

(3) Jalneti is an unfailing remedy for cold, nasal catarrh, sinus, headache and migraine.

(4) Pranayama can be practised more effectively after 'jalneti'.

(2) **Dhauti :** Dhauti can be practised in various ways. But here, only 'vaman dhauti' (kunjal kriya) and 'varisar dhauti' are explained.

Vaman Dhauti :

Take two litres of warm water. Add three or four tea-spoons of salt. Drink six to eight cups of this water. When you feel retching, bend yourself forward and usher the first three fingers deeply into the mouth and give pressure to the hind part of the tongue. Water will be evacuated through vomit.

Continue to usher the fingers into the mouth and vomit as long as all the water in the bowels is evacuated.

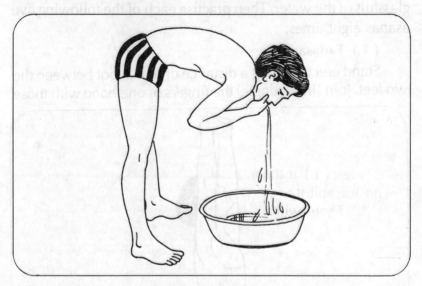

Vaman Dhauti

Note : (1) Vaman dhauti should be practised on an empty stomach.

(2) In this technique, water should be drunk swiftly.

(3) The fingernails should be well manicured.

(4) Food should not be taken for half an hour after vaman dhauti.

(5) Persons suffering from peptic or gastric ulcers, high blood pressure, heart disease and hernia are advised not to practise vaman dhauti.

Repetition : Usually once a week.

Benefits : (1) The digestive organs become active.

(2) Toxic elements, acids and gases are eliminated from the bowels.

(3) Vaman dhauti gives relief in the diseases such as indigestion, chronic cold and asthma.

Varisar Dhauti : Varisar dhauti is an excellent technique to evacuate and cleanse the gastrointestinal tract completely.

Take a bucketful of warm water having some salt in it. Try to keep your mind calm and steady. Swiftly drink two glassfuls of the water. Then practise each of the following five asanas eight times.

(1) Tadasana :

Stand erect keeping a distance of half a foot between the two feet. Join (Intermingle) the fingers of one hand with those

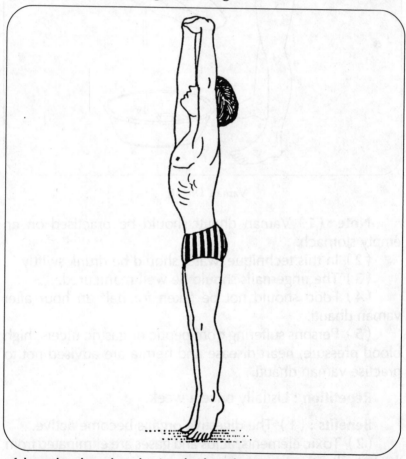

of the other hand and raise the hands up. Raise the heels from the ground and bending the head backwards look at the fingers. Stretch the body upwards. Keep this position for a few seconds and then bring the body to its original position.

Repeat this asana eight times.

(2) Tiryak Tadasana :

First of all, hold the position of Tadasana. Keeping the heels raised from the ground, bend the body first to the right

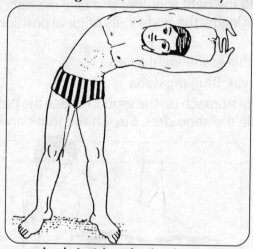

side and then to the left side. The body should be bent at the waist.

Repeat this asana eight times on each side.

(3) Kati Chakrasana :

Stand keeping a distance of two feet between the feet.

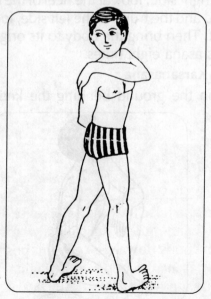

Raise both the arms on the sides of the body to the level of the shoulders. Turn the body by the waist to the right side, bring the left arm to the right shoulder and take the right arm to the back. Then bringing the body to its original position, turn it to the left side.

Repeat this asana eight times.

(4) Tiryak Bhujangasana :

Lie on the stomach on the ground. Place the palms on the ground beside the shoulders. Stretch the trunk and the head

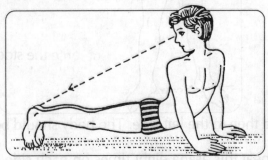

upside with the help of the muscles of the back. Try to minimize the weight on the arms. Now turning the head and the trunk to the right side, look at the heel of the left foot. Then turning the head and the trunk to the left side, look at the heel of the right foot. Then bring the body to its original position.

Repeat this asana eight times.

(5) Udar Karsanasana :

Sit erect on the ground bending the knees. Keep the

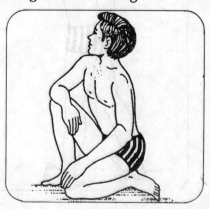

palms on the knees. Lower the left knee to the ground, bend the trunk to the right side as much as possible and look back to the right side. Then come to the original position. Repeat this asana on the other side.

Repeat this asana eight times on both the sides.

Practising the above-mentioned five asanas in the order explained above, sphincter muscles gradually become loose with the result that the saline water drunk through the mouth flows to the anus carrying with it waste food and stool. Drink again two glassfuls of water and practise the above five asanas eight times.

Now go to the toilet. Do not force the stool to come out of the bowels. Keep the muscles of the abdomen relaxed. If the stool does not come out, wait for a minute and then come out of the toilet.

Drink two glassfuls of water again and practising the above-mentioned asanas eight times, go again to the toilet. Never give force to the stool to come out.

Continue this technique (kriya)—drink two glassfuls of water, practise the five asanas and then go to the toilet.

At last, you will be relieved of the stool. In the beginning, the stool will be hard and then the stool mixed with water will come out.

To drink water, to practise asanas and to go to the toilet—if this technique continues in that order, only water would come through the anus. It means that the whole gastrointestinal tract is completely evacuated.

To reach the condition that only water should come through the anus, one has to drink 16 to 20 glasses of water.

As this varisar dhauti is tiring, one who practises it should, after completing it, take rest practising Shavasana for 45 to 60 minutes.

Note : (1) Varisar dhauti should be practised on an empty stomach after evacuating the bowels.

(2) This kriya should be practised under the supervision of an expert.

(3) Persons suffering from peptic or gastric ulcers should not practise varisar dhauti. Persons suffering from high blood pressure or having ailments of the kidney and the blood circulation are advised to practise varisar dhauti under the supervision of an expert.

(4) One who practises varisar dhauti should eat khichadi one hour after the kriya is completed.

Repetition : This kriya should generally be practised once in two or three months. If needs be, 'laghu Shankhprakshalana' kriya should be practised during the days that follow varisar dhauti. In 'laghu Shankhprakshalana' one has to drink two glassfuls of water and practise the abovementioned asanas three times. This kriya helps one to evacuate the bowels and avoid abundant urine.

Benefits : (1) Varisar dhauti gives rest to all the organs of the digestive system with the result that the organs become more active.

(2) Varisar dhauti is an unfailing remedy for chronic constipation, acidity, gas, indigestion and other ailments of the digestive system.

(3) This kriya reduces the quantity of sugar in the blood and so it is useful for those suffering from diabetes.

(3) Nauli : Nauli gives exercise to the abdominal organs.

Stand keeping the distance of about a foot between the two feet. Stoop slightly forward and bend the feet from the knees. Place the palms on the thighs just above the knees. Inhale deeply, then exhale slowly and pull the whole abdominal region back towards the spine. This is known as 'uddiyan bandh'. Now giving pressure on the thighs with the palms push the contracted abdominal muscles downwards. The vertical muscles in the abdomen will now appear forward. This is called 'madhyam nauli'. Maintain this position according to your capacity. Then inhale slowly and relax the abdominal muscles.

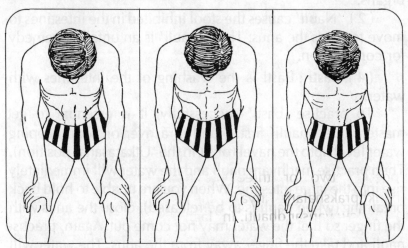

Nauli

During this process, if unequal pressure is given with the palms on the thighs, that is, if more pressure is given on the right thigh, the muscles on the right side will be protruded and if more pressure is given on the left thigh, the muscles on the left side will be protruded. These positions are called 'dakshina nauli' and 'vama nauli' respectively.

After having practised for several days, one can practise these three kinds of 'nauli' which is called 'nauli chalan'.

Note : (1) Practise nauli on an empty stomach after evacuating the bladder and the bowels.

(2) First get mastery over 'uddiyan bandh'. Then gradually learn 'madhyam nauli', 'dakshina nauli', 'vama nauli' and 'nauli chalan' in that order.

(3) During the whole process of 'nauli', 'uddiyana' bandha should continue.

(4) In this technique, a guidance of an expert is necessary.

(5) Persons having pregnancy, high blood pressure, heart disease or severe diseases of the digestive system should not practise nauli.

Repetition : Nauli should be practised every morning.

Benefits : (1) Nauli gives exercise to the abdominal organs.

(2) 'Nauli' causes the stool inhibited in the intestines to move towards the anus. Thus, 'nauli' is an unfailing remedy for constipation.

(**4**) **Basti :** Basti is the washing of the intestines with water.

To practise 'basti' successfully, it is essential to get mastery over 'nauli' first. Stand in a river or pond keeping water level upto the navel (or sit in the 'Utkatasana' position). Then practise madhyam nauli and the water will immediately rise into the large intestine. When you are unable to hold back breathing (when nauli is to be released), close the anus with the finger so that the water may not come out. Again, practise nauli and take the finger away from the anus. The water will rise again into the intestine. If this 'kriya' is practised five to seven times, a good quantity of water will rise into the intestine. If possible, practise 'nauli chalan' and hold back the water for some time. Then come out of the water and go to stools at some proper place.

Note : (1) It is necessary to practise this 'kriya' under the guidance of an expert.

(2) Basti should be practised on an empty stomach early in the morning.

(3) Those who are unable to practise nauli can get the benefits of 'basti' through enema.

Repetition : Once or twice a week.

Benefits : (1) Basti washes away the stool accumulated in the intestine. Thus, 'basti' is a sure remedy for constipation.

(2) Basti activates the intestines.

(**5**) **Tratak :** Tratak is an exercise in which sight is fixed on a particular object.

Sit in the 'Sukhasana' position. Place a burning candle or a small picture or a black dot at a distance of one and a half or two feet away from the face. Look at that object without straining the eyes. Hold back the winking of the eyes. When the eyes are tired or they shed water, shut them and imagine the picture of that object. Open the eyes after some time and practise tratak again. Do this exercise four to five times.

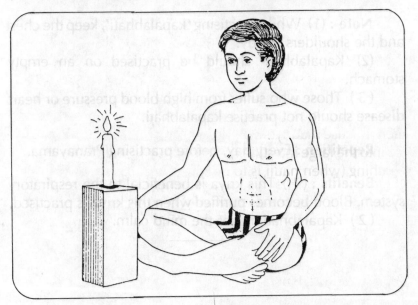

Tratak

Note : (1) If tratak is not performed properly, the eyes may be damaged. It is, therefore, necessary to practise this exercise under the guidance of an expert.

(2) If you practise tratak on the flame of a candle, sit at such a place as is not airy and is dark.

Repetition : Once or twice a day.

Benefits : Tratak strengthens the sight and the eyes become bright. Indirectly, it has a beneficial effect on the brain and the mind.

(6) Kapalabhati : Kapala means 'skull' and 'Bhati' means to 'shine'. Thus, kapalabhati is an exercise the practise of which imparts glow to the skull.

Sit in either the Padmasana or Sukhasana position, keep the body erect. Place the hands on the knees. Inhale and exhale rhythmically and quickly. Then pull in the abdominal muscles and forcefully exhale. Practise this kriya rapidly (60 to 120 times a minute). Then, after about two minutes, stop practising kapalabhati). Let the breathing be normal.

Note : (1) While practising 'kapalabhati', keep the chest and the shoulders steady.

(2) 'Kapalabhati' should be practised on an empty stomach.

(3) Those who suffer from high blood pressure or heart disease should not practise kapalabhati.

Repetition : Every day, before practising Pranayama.

Benefits : (1) This kriya is beneficial to the respiratory system. Blood becomes purified when this kriya is practised.

(2) Kapalabhati makes the mind calm.

4. SITTING POSTURES

1. PADMASANA

'Padma' means lotus. Padmasana acquires its name because when performed this resembles a lotus. This is also known as Kamalasana. This is best suited for meditation and for reciting 'mantras'. This is beneficial to both men and women.

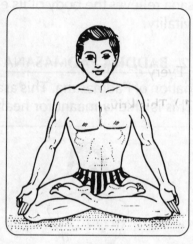

Padmasana

Technique : Sit on the ground. Spread the legs forward and place the right foot on the left thigh and left foot on the right thigh. Some persons like to place first the left foot on the right thigh and then to put the right foot on the left thigh. Either process is right. Let the left hand rest on the left knee and the right hand on the right knee. (See figure.) Let the tips of the thumbs of both the hands touch the tips of the index fingers. Keep the head and the spinal column erect. Keep your eyes close or open. Those who can place only one leg on the thigh should practise this asana daily with zeal. They will be able to perform this asana easily after some practice. Stay in the final position for one or two minutes in the initial stage. Later, increase the time gradually.

29

Advantages : (1) This asana is useful for Japa, Prana-yama, Dharana (Retention or Concentration), Dhyana (Meditation) and Samadhi (Self-realisation).

(2) This asana stimulates the endocrine glands.

(3) This asana is useful to cure diseases like asthma, insomnia and hysteria. It is greatly beneficial to the persons suffering from insomnia.

(4) This asana relieves the body of its excessive fat and it increases the vitality.

2. BADDHA PADMASANA

This is a variation of Padmasana. This asana is not meant for meditation. This is chiefly meant for health-improvement

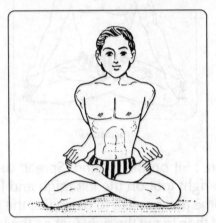

Baddha Padmasana

and for making the body strong. This asana is difficult to perform. Those who are unable to practise this asana should not be disappointed. They should patiently try to accomplish the final position.

Technique : Sit in Padmasana with legs crossed. The heels should touch the lower part of the abdomen. Swing the right arm behind the back of the shoulder and bring the hand near the left hip. Catch the left big toe. Similarly, swing the left arm and hold the right big toe. If you experience difficulty in holding the toes, bend slightly forward and make it convenient to hold the big toes. After catching the toes, sit erect as before and breathe normally. Stay in this position for one or two minutes in the initial stage. Gradually, increase the time till you can stay in the position for ten minutes.

Advantages : (1) In this asana, the weight of the body is borne by the knees and the ankle-joints, so the joints of the legs become strong.

(2) Both the heels of the legs get sufficient exercise.

(3) The continuous practice of this asana helps the person to gradually overcome the weakness of the heart, the lungs, the stomach, the liver and the spine. Moreover, it reduces the pain in the knees and the ankle-joints.

(4) This asana helps to cure ailments like indigestion, flatulence, stomachache, etc.

(5) By practising this asana, one can get all the advantages of Padmasana.

3. PARVATASANA

Parvata means a mountain. This asana is also known as 'Viyogasana', because it involves a special technique of Yoga. Only healthy persons should practise this asana.

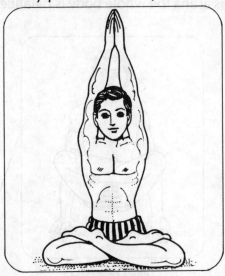

Parvatasana

Technique : Sit in Padmasana. Join the palms of the hands. Stretch the arms vertically up over the head. Some persons perform this asana sitting in the posture of Veera-sana. But the Padmasana posture is better than the Veerasana one. (For Veerasana see page No. 41)

Advantages : (1) As both the arms are kept vertically up in this asana, the 'Prana' is sublimated.

(2) If Suryabheda Pranayama or Anuloma-Viloma Pranayama is practised for fifteen minutes before performing this (Parvatasana) asana, the lungs, the abdomen and the spine become strong and healthy.

(3) This asana gives sufficient exercise to the muscles of the arms.

4. UTTHITA PADMASANA (LOLASANA)

This asana is a variation of Padmasana. In this asana, the body is lifted up with both the hands on the floor. This is the reason why it is called 'Utthita Padmasana' or Lolasana or Dolasana. This asana is more difficult than Padmasana because in this asana the whole body is balanced on both the hands.

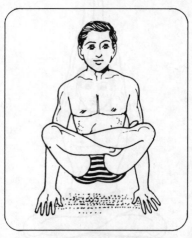

Utthita Padmasana

Technique : Sit in Padmasana. Rest the palms on the floor besides the hips. Slowly raise the trunk without a jerk.

The body should not quiver. Retain the breath in the lungs as long as the body is in the raised position. Exhale when the body is lowered down. While performing this asana, some beginners experience tremor in the hands because of some weakness. But it should not dishearten them. They should practise the asana patiently and with perseverance.

Advantages : (1) This asana strengthens the joints and muscles of the arms.

(2) This asana helps to cure intestinal weakness, constipation, indigestion, dysentery, drowsiness, impurities of tubular channels, etc.

(3) This asana works as an appetiser which is a good characteristic of health.

5. KUKKUTASANA

'Kukkuta' is a Sanskrit word which means a cock. This asana or posture resembles that of a cock and hence the name is Kukkutasana.

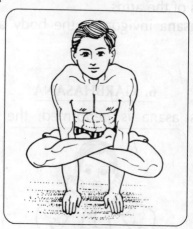

Kukkutasana

Technique : Sit in the Padmasana position. Insert the hands through the gap between the thighs and calves near the knees. Start with the fingers and gradually push the hands up to the elbows. Inhale and raise the body off the floor. Then continue normal breathing. Legs should be raised off the floor up to the level of the elbows. Hands can easily be inserted in the gap if the Padmasana position is slightly raised. Pot-bellied persons will find it difficult to insert the hands in the gap between the calves and the thighs. In the beginning, remain in this position for ten seconds and gradually increase the time to a minute depending upon the age and ability of the aspirant.

Advantages : (1) All the benefits derived from Utthita Padmasana or Lolasana are derived from this asana. The diseases which Utthita Padmasana cures can be cured by this asana also.

(2) This asana is beneficial to those who have worms in their intestines.

(3) This asana is very useful to women as it cures uneasiness, pain in the hips and heaviness caused by menstruation.

(4) This asana gives sufficient exercise to the arms. It stengthens the wrists, the elbows and the shoulders – the three important joints of the arms.

(5) This asana invigorates the body and delights the mind.

6. GARBHASANA

When this asana is performed, the pose achieved

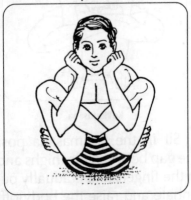

Garbhasana

resembles that of a human foetus in the womb. So this asana is called Garbhasana.

Technique : As in Kukkutasana, insert the hands between the thighs and the calves. Push the arms forward till the elbows can be easily bent. Then hold the lobe of the right ear with the right hand and of the left ear with the left hand. Stay in this position very cautiously to avoid tumbling. The constant practice of this asana will enable you to balance the body on the coccyx (the tail bone). If aspirants experience difficulty in performing this asana in Padmasana position, it should be practised without Padmasana. While performing this asana, let the legs be stretched on the floor. The asana should be performed for 8 to 10 seconds in the beginning. Later, the time of the retention of the asana can be increased to one minute depending on age, ability of the aspirants and benefits expected.

Advantages : (1) This asana helps to cure diseases like colic pain, flatulence, enteritis, chronic fever, constipation, etc.

(2) This asana keeps the abdominal organs trim. It cures gas-trouble and increases the digestion-power.

(3) The abdominal organs, the breast and the joints of the arms and the legs get sufficient exercise through this asana and their ailments disappear.

(4) This asana helps to preserve the semen and the mind begins to have communion with the soul.

7. SIDDHASANA

This asana is performed mostly by the Siddhas – semi divine beings. This is the reason why this asana is called Siddhasana. The main function of this asana is to awaken the power of Kundalini (annular power residing in the mystical circle above the reproductive organs).

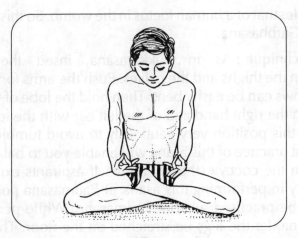

Siddhasana

Technique : Sit on the floor, with legs stretched straight in front. Bend the left leg, hold the left heel, and place it near the perineum. The sole of the left foot should be placed against the right thigh. Now bend the right leg and place the right foot on the left ankle. The heel of the right foot should be placed at the root of the genitals. Place the back of the hands on the knees so that the palms face upward. Join the tip of the thumb and the index finger of each hand. Keep the spine straight and erect. Let the head, the neck and the spine be erect and in the straight line. Look downwards. Bend the neck low so that the chin touches the lower part of the throat.

Advantages : (1) This asana awakens Kundalini Shakti. It purifies all the nadis (tubular channels) in the body through Shaktichalana Mudra.

(2) The asana is good for curing indigestion, chronic fever, dysentery, heart-disease, tuberculosis, asthma, diabetes, etc.

(3) The diseases which can be cured by Padmasana can also be cured by this asana.

(4) This asana is useful for the cure of stiffness in the joints of the loins.

(5) This asana helps the mind to be firm, attentive and alert.

8. SIMHASANA

Simhasana is one of the eighty-four asanas. This asana is also called Bhairavasana. The face posture of this asana, when followed in Vajrasana and Bhadrasana, is known as Simhasana.

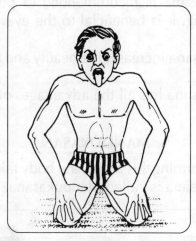

Simhasana

Technique : Bend the legs from the knees and bring them on the backside. Sit on the heels. The heels must be on both the sides of the hips. Let the distance beween the knees be six inches. Place the right palm on the right knee and the left palm on the left knee. Begin exhaling through the nose and the mouth stretching the tongue out from the mouth. Exhaling should be completed as soon as the process of stretching the tongue out from the mouth is completed. Do not breathe now. Keep the trunk erect. Stretch all the facial muscles and widen the eyes in such a way that the face appears frightening. Look straight. Stay in the pose for about six to eight seconds. In the first week, perform this exercise twice a day. Gradually, with practice, increase it to four times a day.

Advantages : (1) This asana is very useful for increasing the power of memory.

(2) This asana works as a medicine for throat-trouble or voice-trouble. It also cures tonsillitis.

(3) It has also a good effect on the respiratory system and on the larynx.

(4) This asana helps to cure all the diseases of the chest and the abdomen.

(5) This asana is recommended to persons suffering from stammering. It is beneficial to the eyes, the nose and the skin.

(6) This asana increases the beauty and the lustre of the face.

(7) This asana has all the advantages of Vajrasana.

9. MANDUKASANA

While performing this asana, the body takes the shape of a frog. So this asana is called Mandukasana.

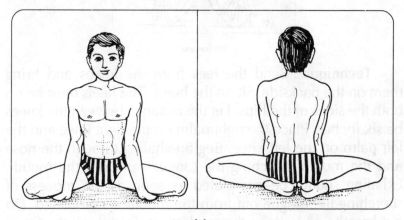

Mandukasana

Technique : Take the legs backwards. Let the feet touch each other. Stretch the knees on both the sides. Rest the hands as shown in the figure. Keep the knees as apart as possible. Keep the trunk straight. Look straight and breathe normally. Remain in this position for eight to twelve seconds. Perform this asana twice in the first week. Later, practise this asana four times.

Advantages : (1) This asana is effective in reducing the weight of the thighs, hips and the abdomen.

(2) This asana strengthens the lower parts of the loins.

(3) This asana increases sexual ability. It removes the defects of the reproductive system of women.

(4) This asana stimulates the digestive system.

(5) The benefits which Padmasana gives can be obtained from this asana also.

10. GOMUKHASANA

'Go' 'गो' means a cow. 'Mukha' 'मुख' means face. When this asana is performed, the performer's posture resembles a cow-head. So it is called Gomukhasana. This is one of the eighty-four asanas.

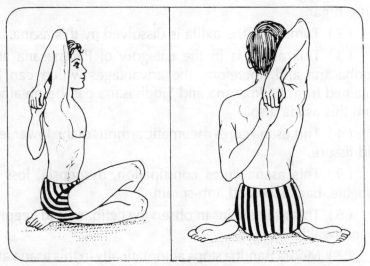

Gomukhasana

Technique : Place the left heel on the left side of the anus. Bend the right leg in such a way that the right knee rests on the left knee and the sole of the right foot touches the lower part of the left thigh. Practice will enable you to bring the right heel to the left thigh. Take the left arm to the back, bend it at the elbow and bring it upward. Now, raise the right arm, bend it at the elbow and take it to the back. Raise the first and the second fingers of the left hand. Lower the first and the second fingers of the right hand. If the fingers slip away, try again for two minutes to bring them to the position. Breathe slowly. Keep the trunk and the head in a straight line. Change the hands in turn. A fat man will find it difficult to perform this asana. But constant practice will enable him to practise the asana comfortably. Practise this asana four times in the first week. Later, gradually increase the frequency and practise it six times. Gradually, increase the duration till the limit of fifteen minutes is reached.

Advantages : (1) As this asana involves all the three Bandhas, Jalandhara Bandha, Uddiyana Bandha and Moola Bandha strongly, Sushumna Nadi naturally gets an abundant flow of oxygen with the result that there is control over the sense organs.

(2) Tumour in the axilla is dissolved by this asana.

(3) This asana is in the category of Padmasana and Siddhasana and, therefore, the advantages which can be obtained from Padmasana and Siddhasana can be obtained from this asana also.

(4) This asana cures rheumatic arthritis of the lower legs and fissure.

(5) This asana cures constipation, dyspepsia, loss of appetite, backache and arm-sprain.

(6) This asana helps in observing celibacy and keeping sound health.

(7) Moola Bandha stops automatically in this asana and so it is very helpful for practising Pranayama.

(8) This asana is useful for longtime meditation.

(9) Joints become flexible and the bones become strong.

(10) This asana strengthens the chest, the lungs and the heart.

11. PADANGUSTHASANA

In ancient time, the persons who lived in Gurukulas and observed celibacy used to practise this asana regularly. With Sheershasana and Sarvangasana, this asana has been given special importance by our sages for the preservation of the semen.

Persons having physical obesity will find it difficult to practise this asana. They may fall on either side while performing this asana. But with constant practice steadiness can be maintained.

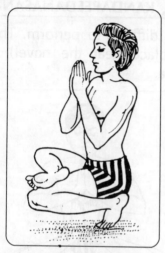

Padangusthasana

Technique : Place the left heel between the anus and the scrotum. Let the weight of the whole body rest on the feet, particularly on the left foot. Place the right foot on the left leg near the knee. Keep the balance while in sitting posture. A bench or a wall can be used as a support in the beginning. Place both the hands on the waist or the thighs, or keep them in the obeisance posture. Retain the breath. Keep the spine erect. Then inhale slowly. Stare at or concentrate on a white or black dot specially kept for this purpose before the eyes. Repeat silently the japa of Ramanama or some gurumantra. Begin practising this asana with 30 seconds and gradually increase it to one minute.

Advantages : (1) As this asana stimulates Veeryanadi, it cures physical disorders like wet-dreams (spermatorrhoea), impotence and diabetes.

(2) The semen is sublimated by practising this asana and it changes into vital energy.

(3) If this asana is practised along with Sheershasana, Sarvangasana and Bhujangasana, it helps one in observing celibacy.

12. KANDAPEEDANASANA

This asana is difficult to perform. This asana presses the Kanda (the place near the navel). So it is called Kandapeedanasana.

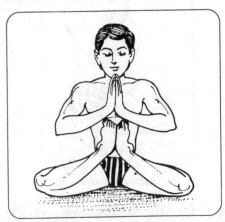

Kandapeedanasana

Technique : Sit on the floor. Bend the legs at the knees. Bring the feet towards the trunk until the heels are close to the perineum, and keep the knees on the floor. Join the palms in front of the chest. Keep the trunk erect. Keep the nose, the palms and the feet in a vertical straight line. Breathe in the normal way. This asana should be practised with caution. Persons whose thighs and calves are heavy will find it difficult to practise this asana. Those having a slim body can perform this asana comfortably.

Advantages : (1) This asana cures all kinds of ailments and disorders of the knees. It also cures arthritis.

(2) It strengthens the calves, arteries and veins.

(3) It stimulates Kundalini Shakti.

(4) This asana is the same as Padmasana or Siddhasana, so it has all the benefits of Padmasana and Siddhasana.

13. VEERASANA

'Veera' means a hero, a warrior. The practice of this asana increases appetite. Those who perform this asana develop the spirit of adventure, enthusiasm and bravery in them.

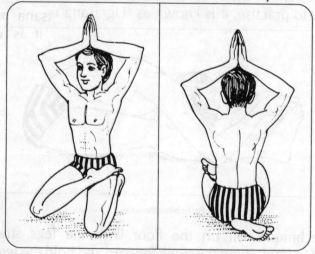

Veerasana

Technique : Sit on the floor. Keep the body erect and the eyes straight. Bend either of the legs at the knee and place the heel below the anus. Bend the other leg at the knee and place it on the thigh of the former leg. Extend the arms forward in line with the shoulders and put them on the head. Keep the loins, the neck and the head in a vertical straight line. Breathe slowly and normally. Hold this position for eight seconds and then assume the posture as in the original position. Then bend the other leg and perform this asana again. The performance of this asana should be repeated six times in a day.

Advantages : (1) All the diseases which Padmasana cures can be cured also by practising this asana. The benefits which Padmasana gives can be obtained from this asana also.

(2) This asana helps in breath-control. So this asana is practised by the best singers of Indian classical music.

(3) This pose is suitable for Pranayama.

14. PASHCHIMOTTANASANA

This asana is also known as 'Ugrasana'. 'Ugra' means 'Shiva'. Lord Shiva is believed to be the god of annihilation. So he is called 'Ugra' or 'the terrible'. As this asana is very difficult to practise, it is known as 'Ugrasana'.

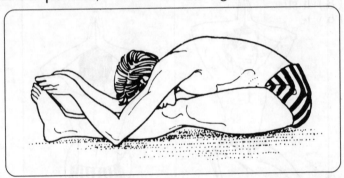

Pashchimottanasana

Technique : Sit on the floor with the legs stretched straight in front. Bend the trunk forward and hold the feet with the thumbs and the first and the middle fingers. Exhale, and bend the trunk lower so that the head rests on the knees. Draw the abdomen in while bending lower. This will make the bending of the trunk easy. While bending bring the head between the arms. The aspirants having flexible spine can touch the knees with the head at the first attempt. Fat persons will find some difficulty in practising this asana. Persons having a weak spine will take a fortnight or a month to accomplish perfection in this asana. Remain in this asana for five seconds. Begin with thirty seconds and gradually increase it to ten minutes.

Advantages : (1) Pashchimottanasana is the foremost of all asanas. Its effect is that the life force flows through the Sushumna nadi and it kindles gastric fire.

(2) The excessive fat around the abdomen is reduced by practising this asana.

(3) It tones up the kidneys, the stomach, the liver and other abdominal organs.

(4) It tones up the intestines and improves digestion.

(5) This asana cures constipation, indigestion, liver-diseases and loss of appetite.

(6) The practice of this asana helps the joints to regain elasticity. It rejuvenates the entire spine.

(7) It makes the body handsome and shapely.

(8) It strengthens the calvic muscles.

(9) It cures hiccough.

15. JANU SHIRASANA

Certain characteristics of this asana are typically the same as those of Pashchimottanasana. In this variation of Pashchimottanasana one leg is extended.

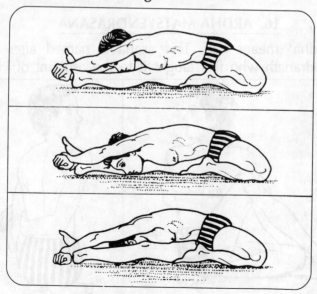

Janu Shirasana

Technique : Sit on the ground. Place the left heel pressing hard near the left groin. Keep the right leg stretched and straight. Hold the right foot with the hands. Exhale and draw the stomach in. Lower the head slowly as shown in the figure. Place the forehead and the chin on the knee. Remain in this position for five to ten seconds. Increase the time gradually. This asana can be practised with the left leg stretched. With constant practice, this asana can be performed for half an hour. Repeat this asana five to six times every day. This asana should be performed after the bowels are emptied. One who practises this asana can practise Pashchimottanasana comfortably.

Advantages : (1) This asana kindles gastric fire and helps digestion.

(2) This asana helps in observing celibacy.

(3) This asana cures kidney troubles.

(4) It cures colic pain.

(5) It awakens the Kundalini which keeps the body free from sluggishness and weakness.

(6) This asana has the same advantages as Pashchimottanasana.

16. ARDHA MATSYENDRASANA

'Ardha' means half. This asana is named after Yogi Matsyendranath who first taught it to the aspirant of Hatha

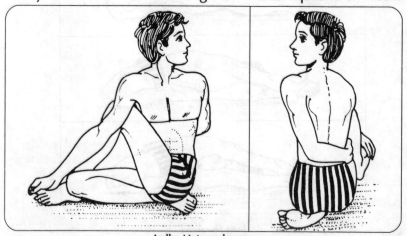

Ardha Matsyendrasana

Yoga. It is said that Matsyendranath was the disciple of Lord Shiva.

Technique : Place the right heel near the anus (buttock) below the testicles. Do not move the heel from this position. Bend the left knee and put the left ankle on the outer side of the right knee. Let the right armpit rest on the outer side of the left thigh. Now push the knee backwards so that it touches the back part of the armpit. Then hold the toe of the left foot with the right hand. Twist the spine slowly exerting force on the joint of the left shoulder. Let the spine be twisted to the left side as far as possible. Turn the head to the left side as far as it can go. Bring it to the line of the left shoulder. Take the left hand backwards and try to hold the right thigh with it. Keep the spine erect. Remain in this position for five to fifteen seconds. Repeat the same in reverse by twisting the spine to the right side. This asana makes the spine twist completely.

Advantages : (1) This asana stimulates appetite.

(2) It awakens the Kundalini and stabilizes Chandranadi.

(3) It makes the spine elastic. It massages the abdominal muscles and organs.

(4) It adjusts and corrects the displacement of the vertebrae, rejuvenating the blood circulation in that part of the body.

(5) It helps one in practising Pashchimottanasana.

17. PURNA MATSYENDRASANA

This asana is easy for those who have practised Ardha Matsyendrasana for some time. Purna Matsyendrasana is a bit difficult to perform in the beginning.

Technique : Sit on the floor with the legs stretched straight in front. Keep the trunk and the head in a vertically straight line. Place the right foot at the root of the left thigh. Place the right heel pressing against the navel. Keep the left foot on the floor behind the right knee. Take the right hand out from under the left knee and with the help of its thumb and

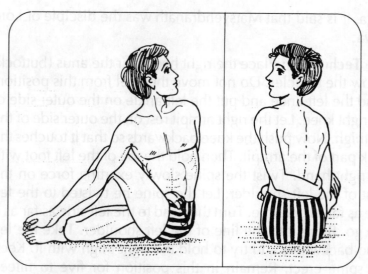

Purna Matsyendrasana

first finger hold the toe of the left foot. Keep the left foot firm in this position. Take your left hand behind the back and keep the head and the body turned to the left side. Twist the waist slightly. Look at the tip of the nose. Breathe in slowly. Retain this position for twenty seconds. The position can be retained for two to three minutes after sufficient practice. This asana gives the maximum benefits when practised on the right and left sides alternately.

Advantages : (1) This asana has all the advantages of Ardha Matsyendrasana.

(2) It alleviates rheumatism.

(3) It stimulates the life energy and cures many diseases.

(4) It supplies fresh blood to the Prananadi. This awakens the Kundalini and the aspirant experiences mental peace and calmness.

(5) This asana is very beneficial to persons suffering from diabetes.

(6) This asana makes the spine flexible and one experiences vigour and vitality of youth.

18. ARDHA VAKRASANA

In this asana, the upper part of the body is twisted and the spine and the back muscles are stretched.

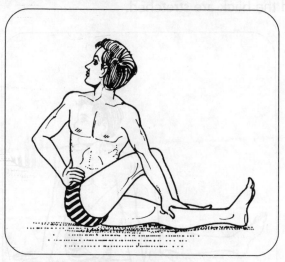

Ardha Vakrasana

Technique : Sit on the floor with the legs stretched in front, keep the legs parallel to each other. Bend the right leg and place it behind the knee of the left leg. Place the left hand on the left knee. Place the right hand on the waist. Keep the trunk straight. Turn backwards on the waist. Remain in this position for six to eight seconds. Inhale slowly. Revert back to the original position. Practise this asana with the other leg stretched, turning the trunk on the other side. Repeat this asana four to five times daily.

Advantages : (1) This asana affects chiefly the waist and the abdominal organs.

(2) It stimulates the spermatozoa glands of men and the uterinal organs of women.

(3) This asana helps in reducing pain in the abdomen and the waist.

(4) It cures constipation and other abdominal ailments.

19. VAKRASANA

In this asana, the upper part of the body is completely turned and twisted. The spine, the muscles of the hands, the legs and the back are stretched.

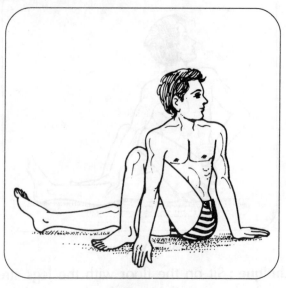

Vakrasana

Technique : Sit on the ground with the legs stretched out. Place the left leg near the right knee, stretching out the left hand behind the back, with the palm of the hand flat resting on the ground. Then press the left knee with the right arm and put the palm on the ground. Keep the waist erect and look as far backward as possible. Practise this asana four to six times a day turning to the left side and to the right side alternately. Gradually, increase the time. The limit is five minutes.

Advantages : (1) This asana strengthens the spine and activates the nerves.

(2) The mouth of the Sushumna opens and Kundalini Shakti is sublimated.

(3) This asana invigorates the muscles of the loins.

(4) Purna Vakrasana bestows all the benefits gained by performing Ardha Vakrasana.

20. AKARNA DHANURASANA

This asana resembles a strung bow. So it is called Akarna Dhanurasana. There are two methods of practising this asana.

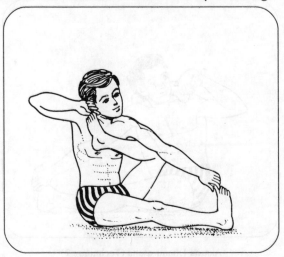

Akarna Dhanurasana (Technique 1)

Technique 1 : Sit on the ground. Stretch the legs in front. Hold the toe of the right foot with the left hand. Hold the left leg with the right hand and try to stretch the right elbow backwards as far as possible. Now bend the left leg slowly. Bring the left foot to the chin and the left knee to the left armpit. This position will bring the thigh close to the abdomen. Hold the breath and then exhale slowly. Repeat the pose on the other leg. Gradually, increase the time duration of holding the posture maximum to five minutes.

Technique 2 : Sit on the floor with the legs stretched in front. Lift the left leg up and hold it with the left hand behind the neck in such a way that the thumb remains forward near the ankle and the fingers behind the thumb. The weight of the leg falls on the palm. Then with the right hand hold the upper part of the left foot with its heel. Place the shin on the neck. Turn the neck towards the right side. Stretch the left arm and hold the right toes. At the same time, lift the right arm up and hold the left toes. Look to the right side. Then release the legs slowly. Repeat this asana with the other leg. Gradually, increase the time of holding the posture maximum to five minutes.

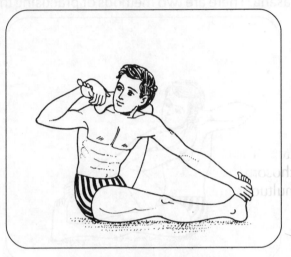

Akarna Dhanurasana (Technique 2)

Advantages : (1) The practice of this asana gives full exercise to the joints of the hands and the legs, the joints and the muscles of the neck and the spine. It revitalizes them.

(2) It tones up the chest and the abdominal organs.

(3) Those who suffer from asthma, tuberculosis and cough get relief if they practise this asana.

(4) As this asana strengthens the lungs, the chest is expanded and it gets the capacity to hold air.

(5) This asana cures the pain in the loins, tonsillitis, indigestion, constipation, the tumour in the armpit, gout, pain in the legs, etc.

(6) This asana alleviates women's complaints of irregular menstruation, the disorders of ovary and pain in the lower part of the abdomen.

5. SUPINE POSTURES

1. SHAVASANA

Shavasana is also called 'Mrutasana'. This asana is very useful for meditation, Pranayama, Japa, etc. This asana should precede other asanas. It should be performed at intervals and also at the end. This asana relaxes the muscles and the blood vessels. Though this asana appears simple, it is one of the most difficult to master. The practice of this asana aims at releasing the mind from the body. This asana is Yogic relaxation in the shortest possible time. Relaxation of the body and the mind is necessary in this modern age of commotion and materialism. Shavasana has been accepted as a remedy for psychosomatic diseases caused on account of competitive and tumultuous life.

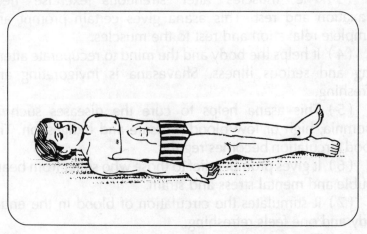

Shavasana

Technique : Lie flat on the back. Place the hands a little away from the thighs with the palms up. Keep the eyes and the fists slightly closed. Stretch the legs out. Keep the heels together and the toes apart. Now close the eyes and breathe very slowly. Begin by consciously and gradually relaxing each part and each muscle of the body : feet, calves, knees, thighs, abdomen and hips. Then relax the muscles of the back, chest, arms, fingers, neck, head and face in that order. Inhale and exhale slowly and deeply. Relax the brain during exhalation. Direct your attention to the breathing, to the soul and to God. Retain the meditation for ten to fifteen minutes. In this posture, one finds true relaxation and experiences rest, peace and plenitude. Those who suffer from excessive mental stress or heart-disease must practise only Shavasana regularly every day.

Advantages : (1) Posture and meditation are co-ordinated in Shavasana. Shavasana pacifies the body and the mind.

(2) In Shavasana, all parts of the body – skin, muscles and nerves – are relaxed.

(3) The muscles after strenuous exercise need relaxation and rest. This asana gives certain prompt and complete relaxation and rest to the muscles.

(4) It helps the body and the mind to recuperate after a long and serious illness. Shavasana is invigorating and refreshing.

(5) This asana helps to cure the diseases such as insomnia, high or low blood pressure and indigestion. The blood circulation becomes regular.

(6) It gives prompt relief to those who suffer from heart-trouble and mental stress and strain.

(7) It stimulates the circulation of blood in the entire body and one feels refreshing.

(8) The constant practice of this asana helps one to control anger.

In view of the benefits mentioned above, every aspirant of Yoga should perform this asana regularly every day.

2. EKAPADA UTTANASANA

This asana gives sufficient exercise to the abdominal muscles. This asana is to be performed with one leg at a time and then changing it to the other leg.

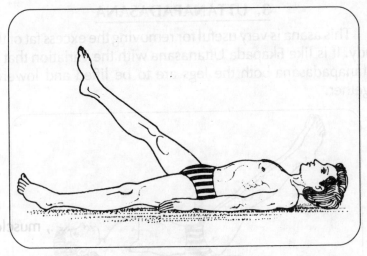

Ekapada Uttanasana

Technique : Lie on the back. Keep the heels together. Put the hands on the floor by the side of the body. Stretch one of the feet forward and loosen the other leg. Inhale slowly. Slowly lift the tight leg up. Hold the breath. Remain in this position for six to eight seconds. Then slowly lower the leg without jerk and exhale. Take rest for six to eight seconds and practise this exercise with the other leg. In the beginning, this asana should be practised four times with each leg. After practice, one can practise this asana six times with each leg. This asana being easy should be performed regularly by a student of Yoga.

Advantages : (1) This asana relieves stomach pains and tones up the liver, the spleen and the kidneys.

(2) It cures indigestion, gas-trouble and intestinal disorders.

(3) It reduces abdominal obesity.

(4) It relieves pain during menstrual periods.

(5) It removes swelling in the legs, tones up the blood circulation in the legs and relieves pain in the knees and the lower parts of the legs.

(6) It has a beneficial effect on the upper part of the body (thorax). It strengthens the lungs.

3. UTTANAPADASANA

This asana is very useful for removing the excess fat of the body. It is like Ekapada Uttanasana with the variation that in Uttanapadasana both the legs are to be lifted and lowered together.

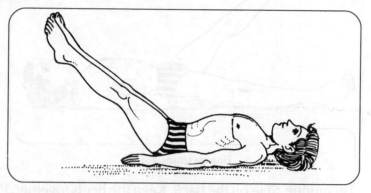

Uttanapadasana

Technique : Lie flat on the back. Keep the arms by the side of the body. Keep the heels and the feet together. Inhale slowly. Then lift the legs up slowly. Retain this position for six to eight seconds. Hold the breath. Bring the legs slowly down on the floor. Exhale. Take rest for six to eight seconds and repeat the same. In the beginning, practise this asana four times a day and gradually increase it to five or six times a day.

Advantages : (1) This asana gives sufficient exercise to every muscle of the abdomen. The abdominal muscles are strengthened and the digestive system functions efficiently.

(2) It tones up the pancreas and alleviates indigestion and constipation.

(3) This asana reduces the fat in the body.

(4) This asana is beneficial to those who suffer from backache and pains of the loins and thighs. Moreover, it is a boon to those who suffer from the discomfort caused by intestinal worms.

(5) It rejuvenates the spinal nerves and the brain cells, strengthens the muscles and activates them.

(6) This asana is a good remedy for piles in the initial stage.

(7) This asana cures hiccough, pain in the thighs, belching, constipation and helps expelling the wind at the anus.

(8) It is an introduction to Sarvangasana.

4. PAVANAMUKTASANA

As its name suggests, this asana gives relief from excess wind in the belly. This asana can be performed by raising one leg or both the legs.

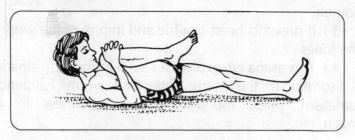

Pavanamuktasana (with one leg)

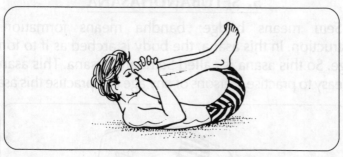

Pavanamuktasana (with both the legs)

Technique : Lie flat on the back. Keep the heels of both the legs together. Inhale deeply and bend the right knee towards the stomach and hold it with both the hands. Raise the head above the ground and bring the chin closer to the knee so that it touches the knee-cap. Exhale and press the muscles of the right abdomen with the right thigh. Keep the stomach pressed till the breath is suspended. This asana is called 'Dakshina Pavanamuktasana'. If this asana is performed with the left leg, it is called 'Vama Pavanamuktasana'. Practise this exercise with both the legs together. This is called 'Purna Pavanamuktasana'. While holding the legs with both the hands, exhale and control the breathing. Then slowly begin inhaling while stretching the legs out. (Women are advised not to practise this asana after conception.)

Advantages : (1) Pavanamuktasana is the best natural way to get rid of foul gases.

(2) It reduces obesity of the body and the fat around the abdomen.

(3) It prevents heart-trouble and improves the working of the lungs.

(4) This asana cures diseases such as gas, constipation, the disorders of the uterus, intestinal worms, appendix, rheumatism, piles, blood-impurities, windiness in the stomach, etc.

5. SETUBANDHASANA

Setu means bridge; bandha means formation or construction. In this asana, the body is arched as if to form a bridge. So this asana is called Setubandhasana. This asana is very easy to practise. Persons of any age can practise this asana.

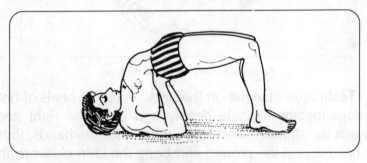

Setubandhasana

Technique : Lie on the back. Bend both the knees. Raise the loins and the thighs upward. Keep the back of the head, the neck and the shoulders firmly on the floor. Breathe normally. Remain in this position for six to eight seconds. Then take some rest and repeat the exercise. Practise this exercise four times a day in the beginning. Later, practise it six times a day.

Advantages : (1) This asana cures the diseases of the loins and the thighs.

(2) It gives exercise to the shoulders, the neck, the elbows and the hands. The constant practice of this asana strengthens these parts of the body.

(3) It expels excess of gases and cures indigestion.

(4) This asana makes the spine flexible and active.

6. TOLANGULASANA

When this asana is performed, the body takes the shape of scales. So it is called Tolangulasana.

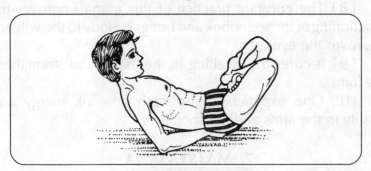

Tolangulasana

Technique : Lie with the foot-lock as in Padmasana. Place your hands, palms upward, under the middle part of the hips. If it is difficult to place the palms under the hips, lift the body up with the help of the elbows and rest. Thus, the body will remain supported on the elbows and the hips. Hold the breath as long as possible. Then exhale slowly. Keep the eyes open and the body stretched. Breathe normally. Bend the neck forward and fix the eyes on the navel. Retain the posture for half a minute to begin with, and progressively, but quite slowly, increase the duration maximum to three minutes depending on individual age, strength and benefits desired. Practise this asana five to ten times.

Advantages : (1) This asana relieves foul gases accumulated in the stomach.

(2) This asana makes the vertebral column elastic and flexible.

(3) The abdominal tension pushes down all faecal matter to the end of the passage of the colon.

(4) It stimulates blood circulation in the muscles and the nerves of the arms and the hands which are incidently toned up and strengthened.

(5) It strengthens and enlarges the rib-box.

(6) It increases the elasticity of the spine and tones up the nervous system.

(7) It cures diseases such as constipation, dysentery, asthma, tuberculosis and diabetes.

(8) The constant practice of this asana improves the functioning of the soundbox and brings melody to the voice. It improves the eyesight.

(9) It cures the swelling in the thighs and strengthens the loins.

(10) One experiences the fresh flow of energy and vitality in the arms and the shoulders.

7. MATSYASANA

This asana is known as Matsyasana because in this asana, with the help of Plavini Pranayama, one can float on the surface of water,like a fish.'Matsya'is the Sanskrit word for fish. This asana is not very difficult to perform. Some practice will enable one to perform this asana easily. This asana is very useful for concentration, meditation and self-realization. There are three techniques to perform this asana.

Technique 1 : Lie flat on the back. Start with the Padmasana pose with the right leg on the left thigh and the left leg on the right thigh. Lock the forearms and rest your head on

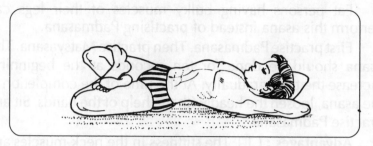

Matsyasana (Technique 1)

on them. Breathe normally. This is the first technique of practising Matsyasana.

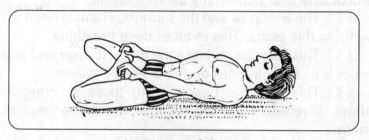

Matsyasana (Technique 2)

Technique 2 : Sit in Padmasana and then lie flat on the back. Hold the left toe with the right hand and the right toe with the left hand.

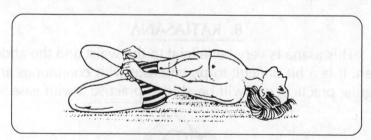

Matsyasana (Technique 3)

Technique 3 : Sit in Padmasana and lie flat on the back. Slide the head backwards in such a way that the crown of the head and the hips would support the body. Between the head and the hips, an arch is formed similar to a bridge. Now stretch your arms forward and hold the toes with the fingers. In this technique, the neck is pulled in such a way that it gives the body the shape of an arch.

Fat persons having bulky muscles of their legs can perform this asana instead of practising Padmasana.

First practise Padmasana. Then practise Matsyasana. This asana should be done for ten seconds at the beginning. Increase the time gradually. At the time of the completion of the asana, loosen the head with the help of the hands. Sit and practise Padmasana.

Advantages : (1) The stiffness in the neck-muscles and the dullness around the throat-muscles caused by Sarvangasana can be alleviated by practising Matsyasana immediately after performing Sarvangasana.

(2) The windpipe and the soundbox remain open while practising this asana. This induces deep breathing.

(3) This exercise enlarges the thoracic cage and allows deeper breathing. It tones up the digestive system.

(4) This asana is beneficial to those suffering from asthma. It removes the disorders of the entire respiratory system.

(5) It activates the spinal column and the muscles of the back.

(6) It stimulates the facial nerves and blood vessels thus brightens up the face.

8. KATIASANA

This asana is very beneficial to the waist and the abdomen. It is a bit difficult to practise but with continuous and regular practice, one will be able to practise it with ease.

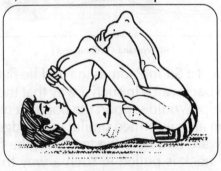

Katiasana

Technique : Lie flat on the back. Raise both the legs up. Now hold the left toe with the left hand and the right toe with the right hand. Then straighten both the legs. Inhale deeply. The head and the waist should be firmly attached to the floor. Remain in this position for about ten seconds and then revert to the original position. In the beginning, practise this asana four times daily. Later, it can be practised six times a day.

Advantages : (1) This asana cures all the diseases of the waist.

(2) It is a sure remedy for colic pain.

(3) It strengthens the lungs and the shoulders.

(4) It stimulates the blood circulation in the heart, purifies the blood and prevents heart-troubles.

9. SUPTABHADRASANA

This asana is also called 'Suptagorakshasana'. Japa, Pranayama, Dhyana (Meditation) and other activities can be performed easily in this asana. This can be performed in two different postures.

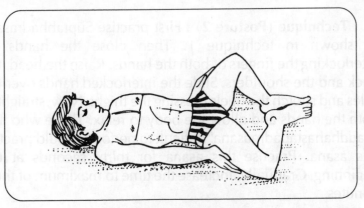

Suptabhadrasana (Technique 1)

Technique (Posture 1) : Bend the right leg at the knee and join the heel in front of the right side of the genitals. Similarly, bend the left leg at the knee and join the heel in front of the left side of the genitals. Let the soles touch each other. Then lie flat on the back. Now, lie in such a way as the heels do not touch the part close to the genitals. While performing this exercise, the soles of both the feet should be in constant touch with each other. Now, spread the arms sideways and place the hands on the thighs and press them down quite gently. Both the arms should remain straight. Do this exercise for thirty seconds in the beginning and gradually increase the time to maximum of fifteen minutes.

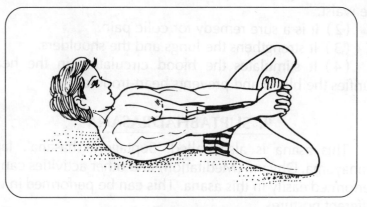

Suptabhadrasana (Technique 2)

Technique (Posture 2) : First practise Suptabhadrasana as shown in technique 1. Then close the hands by interlocking the fingers of both the hands. Raise the head, the neck and the shoulders. Slide the interlocked hands over the soles and stretch the heels pressing the thighs. Now, straighten both the hands and allow the body to relax. Those who find 'Baddhahastapadmasana' difficult to perform should practise this asana. Practise this asana for thirty seconds at the beginning. Gradually, increase the time to maximum of three minutes.

Advantages : (1) This asana stimulates the blood circulation with the result that the internal glands function properly.

(2) It strengthens the heart. The heart beats normally even if one works strenuously.

(3) As the spine remains erect in this asana, the activities like Japa, Pranayama, Meditation, etc. can be done easily.

(4) It sublimates Kundalini Shakti.

(5) As this asana makes every system of the body much more active, the body becomes healthy and the mind cheerful.

(6) The second technique of Suptabhadrasana strengthens the joints and the muscles of the arms and the legs.

(7) This asana is of the same category of Padmasana, Matsyasana and Padmadolasana, so it has all the benefits of those asanas. It can cure all such diseases as are cured by the asanas mentioned above.

10. VIPARITAKARANI MUDRA OR VILOMASANA

Mudras are the developed forms of asanas. Holding the body in particular postures in order to control the sense

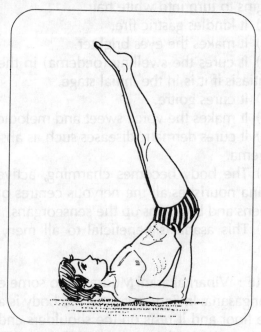

Viparitakarani Mudra

organs is of prime importance in asanas, whereas in Mudras, main thrust is given on Prana, the root of human life. Our scriptures speak very high about the achievement of Mudras in this world. He who practises them only for a period of three hours every day conquers time.

Technique : Lie flat on the back and inhale as in complete Yogic breathing. Exhale and raise the legs and hips with the help of the arms and hold the hips in the hands so that the body is supported on the elbows. Gaze at the toes. This exercise is called Viparitakarani because, when practised, the body takes up an inverted position. Some people consider Sheershasana to be 'Viparitakarani Mudra'. In the beginning, this posture should be maintained for a minute only. Increase the time to ten minutes – a limit to be attained gradually.

Advantages : (1) This asana prevents the formation of wrinkles on the face. It slackens the process in which black hair begins to turn into white hair.

(2) It kindles gastric fire.

(3) It makes the eyes brighter.

(4) It cures the swelling (oedema) in the leg. It cures elephantiasis if it is in the initial stage.

(5) It cures goitre.

(6) It makes the voice sweet and melodious.

(7) It cures dermatic diseases such as abscess, pimples and eczema.

(8) The body becomes charming, active and strong. This asana nourishes all the nervous centres of the brain. It strengthens and brightens up the senseorgans.

(9) This asana is beneficial to all men, women and children.

Note : 'Viparitakarani Mudra' is, to some extent, similar to Sarvangasana. In Sarvangasana, the body is at right angles with the floor and it rests on the shoulders and the neck. In 'Viparitakarani', the lower part of the trunk is curved up inclining to the ground.

11. SARVANGASANA

This is one of the most important asanas. Sarvangasana literally means 'all parts pose'. When this asana is practised, all the parts of the body are exercised. So it is called Sarvangasana.

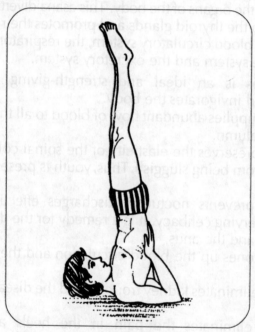

Sarvangasana

Technique : Lie on the back with the body fully stretched. Inhale as in complete Yogic breathing. Slowly raise the legs together. Then raise the legs, the hips and the trunk in a continuous movement until they attain a vertical position. Support the back on two sides with both the hands. Keep the elbows on the ground. Let the shoulders and the neck touch the ground. Keep the body steady. Keep the legs raised straight up. Breathe normally. Look at the toes of the feet. Bend the legs towards the head. Relax the body and bring the legs back to the ground without jerking the spine. In this asana, the weight of the entire body is borne by the shoulders. Concentrate your mind on the thyroid gland in the lower part of the throat. This asana can be practised twice a day–in the morning and in the evening. This asana should be followed by Matsyasana to derive all the benefits of Sarvangasana. Practise this asana for two minutes in the beginning gradually increasing the time to the limit of half an hour.

Advantages : (1) Healthy thyroid means healthy functioning of all the organs of the body. This asana diverts the flow of blood into the thyroid glands and promotes their health. It tones up the blood circulatory system, the respiratory system, the digestive system and the excretory system.

(2) This is an ideal and strength-giving asana. It energises and invigorates the body.

(3) It supplies abundant flow of blood to all the roots of the spinal column.

(4) It preserves the elasticity of the spinal column and prevents it from being sluggish. Thus, youth is preserved for a long time.

(5) It prevents nocturnal discharges effectively and helps in observing celibacy. It is a remedy for the diseases of the genitals and the anus.

(6) It tones up the blood circulation and the digestive system.

(7) It eliminates kidney troubles and the diseases of the bladder.

(8) It eliminates the pain in the heels and other disorders of the feet.

(9) It is beneficial to those who suffer from anaemia and leprosy.

(10) It tones up the functioning of the nose and the ears. It purifies blood.

(11) Women can safely practise this asana. This asana eliminates the disorders of the ovary.

(12) It awakens the Kundalini and stimulates gastric juices.

(13) It eliminates the longtime diseases of the intestines like indigestion.

(14) If there is a shortage of time, Sarvangasana, Matsyasana, Shirshasana and Pashchimottanasana can keep you in perfect health.

12. HALASANA

Halasana is so named because the posture assumed in doing this asana resembles a plough, for which Hala is the Sanskrit word.

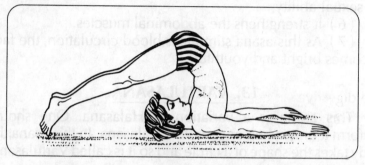

Halasana

Technique : Lie flat on the back with the arms stretched by the side of the body, palms flat on the ground. Place the legs together and keep them straight. Inhale and raise the legs up slowly. Inhaling and the raising of the legs up should be simultaneous. Do not bend the knees. Do not raise the arms. Do not bend the back. When you are in Sarvangasana posture, exhale and at the same time begin lowering the legs over the head till the toes touch the ground. Keep the knees together and straight. Keep the thighs and the legs straight. Breathe normally till the asana is completed. Do not breathe through the mouth. Keep the eyes closed or open. See that the legs remain straight. Let the chin touch the throat. Hold this position for eight to ten seconds. Then slowly raise the legs and without giving them a jerk bring them to the ground in the original position.

Advantages : (1) This asana nourishes the blood vessels of the spinal column, the muscles of the back, vertebrae and the nerves which pass by both the sides of vertebrae.

(2) It makes the spine flexible and elastic. As a result, a habitual aspirant of Halasana becomes very agile, alert and vigorous.

(3) It eliminates muscular rheumatism, lumbar pain, sprain and neuritis.

(4) It cures constipation, gastric trouble and reduces irregular contraction and expansion of the liver and the spleen.

(5) According to the Yoga textbooks, this asana, tones up sexual ability.

(6) It strengthens the abdominal muscles.

(7) As this asana stimulates blood circulation, the face becomes bright and youthful.

13. VARTULASANA

This asana is a variation of Halasana. One should perform it only when one masters Halasana. In this asana, the body takes the shape of a circle and so it is called Vartulasana.

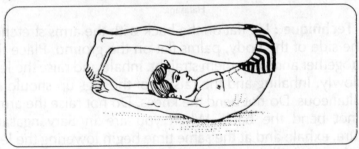

Vartulasana

Technique : Lie on the back and first practise Halasana. Then slowly raise the arms and hold the toes with the hands. Do not give a jerk to the body while doing this exercise. Hold this position for eight to ten seconds. Then slowly raise the legs up and without giving the body a jerk bring them back to the ground in the original position. Then place the arms straight by the sides of the hips.

Advantages : (1) This asana increases youthful energy because it invigorates the sexual organs. This asana is helpful for curing impotence.

(2) It reduces fat around the loins.

(3) It gives enough exercise to the blades of the shoulders.

(4) It enhances the benefits acquired by Sarvangasana.

(5) It has all the benefits of Halasana.

6. ABDOMINAL POSTURES

1. ARDHA SHALABHASANA

'Shalabha' is the Sanskrit word for locust. 'Shalabh-asana' is so called because, while performing it, the body assumes a posture which resembles a locust. When this asana is practised with one leg, it is called 'Ardha Shalabhasana'.

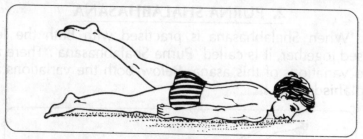

Ardha Shalabhasana

Technique : Lie on the stomach with the face down on the ground. Stretch both the arms beside the body and clench the fists lightly. The hands can also be placed under the thighs. Inhale and retain the breath till the completion of the asana. Pull the body and raise either of the legs by about 30 cms off the ground. Raise the leg as high as possible. Stretch the soles of the feet. Hold this position for five to thirty seconds. Then slowly bring the leg down on the ground. Exhale very slowly. Repeat this exercise with the other leg. This asana can be repeated six to seven times.

Advantages : (1) As far as the spinal bend is concerned, this asana is inverse to Pashchimottasana. This asana gives twist backwards to the spine.

(2) Bhujangasana develops the (half) upper part of the trunk, while Shalabhasana develops the remaining lower part of the trunk.

(3) It is very useful in extricating waste matter accumulated in the intestines.

(4) It cures lumbar pain and reduces excessive fat formed around the knees, the thighs, the waist and the abdomen.

(5) It gives good exercise to the abdomen. The kidney, the liver, etc. become active. It strengthens the ovary.

(6) It cures constipation, gas-trouble, indigestion, dysentery, acidity and other abdominal disorders.

(7) The practice of this asana counters tendencies to piles. It removes the aches of the soles of the feet and cures the disease of the appendix.

2. PURNA SHALABHASANA

When Shalabhasana is practised with both the legs raised together, it is called 'Purna Shalabhasana'. There are two variations of this asana. Below both the variations are explained.

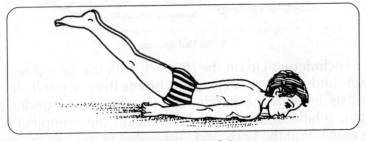

Purna Shalabhasana (Technique 1)

First Variation (Technique) : Lie on the stomach with the forehead touching the ground. Stretch the arms beside the body. Keep the thumbs and the index fingers on the ground and clench the fists. Stiffen the body and raise the legs as high as possible. Stretch the soles of the feet. Pull the legs, the thighs and the lower part of the abdomen up. Hold this position for five to thirty seconds and rest the breath. Bring the legs down slowly and then exhale smoothly.

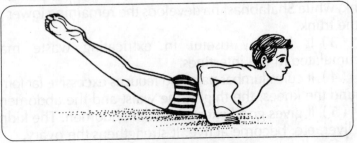

Purna Shalabhasana (Technique 2)

Second Variation (Technique) : Resume the position of the first variation of Shalabhasana. Then raise the head. Place the arms on the floor by the side of the chest, the palms facing the floor.

Advantages : (1) This asana brings pressure on the abdomen and strengthens the muscles of the abdomen, thighs and legs.

(2) It tones up the abdominal organs such as the gall bladder, the stomach, the spleen and the bladder, and cures abdominal disorders.

(3) In increases gastric fire and improves digestion.

(4) It cures oedema.

(5) It cures tumour.

(6) It gives new energy to the throat.

(7) It cures strangury, diabetes and other disorders of the kidney.

(8) The practice of this asana removes the pain in the ovary which women experience during menstruation.

(9) It cures the diseases of the lungs.

(10) It cures dropsy (ascites) for ever and has a beneficial effect on the fistula in its initial stage.

3. BHUJANGASANA

'Bhujanga' means a serpent. In the pose of Bhujangasana, one imitates a cobra reared up on its caudal support and the hood fully expanded. So this asana is called Bhujangasana.

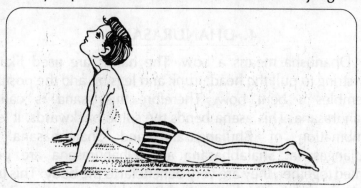

Bhujangasana

Technique : Lie on the floor with the face downwards.

Relax all the muscles of the body. Place the palms on the ground underneath the shoulders. Slowly raise the head and the trunk like the hood of a serpent. Bend the spine backwards. Stretch the feet backwards so that the toes touch the ground. This will stretch well the muscles of the back and the shoulders. There will be strain on the abdomen. Hold the breath and hold this position for six to eight seconds. Then exhale and bring the head to its original position. When you first lie on the ground,keep the chin touching the chest. Hold the breath till the head remains in the raised position. Then exhale slowly. Practise this asana five to six times.

Advantages : (1) This asana removes spinal pain and cures other spinal disorders.

(2) This asana exerts pressure on the internal organs of the abdomen. It pushes waste matter to the anus and thus cures constipation and increases the heat in the body.

(3) It strengthens the ovary and the uterus. It removes the disorders related to menstruation. This asana stimulates blood circulation in the uterus with the result that delivery becomes natural and easy.

(4) It exercises the spine properly, activates the abdominal organs and removes abdominal pain.

(5) It develops the chest, the neck, and other parts of the head. It makes the body shapely.

4. DHANURASANA

Dhanusha means a bow. The hands are used like a bowstring to pull the head, trunk and legs up and the posture resembles a bent bow. Therefore this asana is called Dhanurasana. This asana bends the spine backwards. It is a combination of Bhujangasana and Shalabhasana. If Bhujangasana, Shalabhasana and Dhanurasana are performed together, they are very beneficial to the body. This trio works contrary to Halasana and Pashchimottanasana which bend the spine forward.

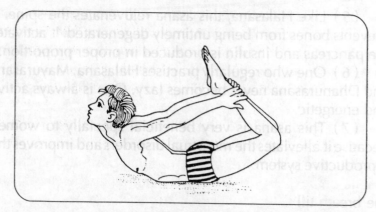

Dhanurasana

Technique : Lie prone on the floor on the stomach, face downwards. Relax the muscles. Keep the arms resting alongside the body. Bend the legs at the knees. Raise the arms and hold the ankles with the hands. Raise the chest and the head. Fill the lungs with air. Straighten and stiffen the hands. Stiffen the legs also. The body now assumes the posture of a convex arch. If you lift the legs up, you can raise the chest. Hold the breath. Then exhale slowly. Attempt to keep the knees together.

In this asana, the abdomen supports the whole body. So practise this asana when the stomach is empty. The body in Dhanurasana pose gets good exercise if it is lightly rocked from left to right and forward and backward. Stay in this position as long as possible. It can be practised five to six times.

Advantages : (1) This asana gives a good massage to the abdomen so it cures prolonged constipation, dyspepsia and other disorders of the stomach.

(2) It cures spinal hump and rheumatism of the legs, the knees and the hands.

(3) It reduces fat. It activates the intestines and increases the digestive power. It nourishes all the abdominal organs by supplying blood to them.

(4) This asana is a blessing to those who suffer from gas and other intestinal disorders.

(5) Like Halasana, this asana rejuvenates the spine. It prevents bones from being untimely degenerated. It activates the pancreas and insulin is produced in proper proportion.

(6) One who regularly practises Halasana, Mayurasana and Dhanurasana never becomes lazy. One is always active and energetic.

(7) This asana is very beneficial specially to women because it alleviates the menstrual disorders and improves the reproductive system.

5. MAKARASANA

'Makara' means a crocodile. In this asana, the body assumes the shape of a crocodile floating in water. So, this asana is called Makarasana.

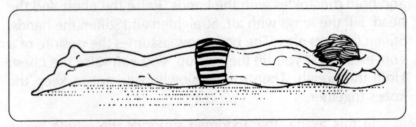

Makarasana

Technique : Lie on the ground face down, the chest touching the ground and both legs stretched out. Let the upper parts of the feet touch the ground. Keep the heels upwards. Raise the arms and put them in front of the head and hold the middle part of the left upper arm with the right hand and the middle part of the right upper arm with the left hand. Keep the head downwards and close the eyes. The head will rest on the arms. The parts of the arms from the elbows to shoulders, the abdomen, the thighs and the upper parts of the feet will touch the ground in a straight line. Relax the body while practising this asana. Breathe deeply and meditate on God.

Advantages : (1) It eradicates the fatigue and gives relaxation to all the parts of the body.

(2) Though the process of practising this asana is inverse to that of practising Shavasana, the aim of both the asanas is the same : to give relaxation and complete rest to the body.

(3) Like Shavasana, this asana is useful to those whose spine or back is injured.

6. VIPARITA MATSYASANA

This is a reverse posture of Matsyasana, hence it is called Viparita Matsyasana. This is called Supta Padmasana also.

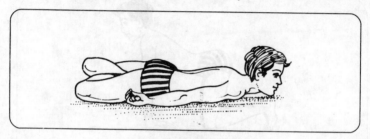

Viparita Matsyasana

Technique : Lie on the left side of the body. Place both legs in the position of Padmasana. Then lie on the chest and abdomen. Bend the neck to the back and put the chin on the ground. Hold the toes with the thumbs and index fingers of the hands. Inhale slowly. Hold this position for eight to ten seconds. Gradually, increase the time to the limit of ten minutes.

Advantages : (1) This asana broadens the chest and strengthens the lungs. It gives the maximum benefit to the spine with the minimum effort.

(2) The regular practice of this asana exercises the joints of the neck as well as the large and small joints of the body. It tones up the muscles.

(3) It eliminates the diseases such as constipation, gas-trouble, indigestion, cold, tuberculosis, asthma and dysentery.

7. HAND-POSTURES

1. MAYURASANA

'Mayura' means a peacock. This asana is a straight plane with the forearms as levers. When this asana is performed, the body assumes the posture which resembles a peacock, which explains the Sanskrit name Mayurasana. Compared with other asanas, this asana is difficult to practise. Physical fitness is a prerequisite to practise this asana. To gymnasts this asana is easy.

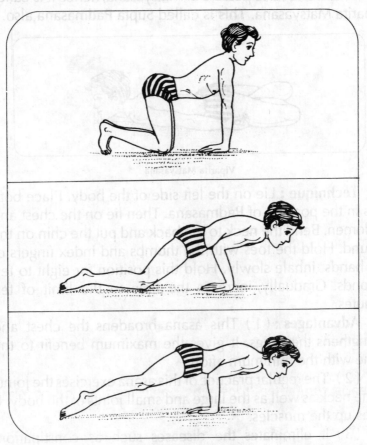

Preparation for Mayurasana

Technique : Kneel on the floor with the knees slightly apart. Support the legs on the feet. Invert the palms and place them between the knees. There should be a distance of three to four cms between the palms. The little fingers should be placed together pointing towards the feet. The thumbs should firmly press the ground. Keep both the hands steady and firm. Then slowly bring the elbows close to the abdomen just under the navel. Rest the diaphragm on the elbows. The elbows are placed together to provide a suitable fulcrum on which the horizontal body could rest. This is the first stage of Mayurasana.

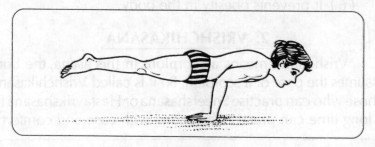

Mayurasana

Now, stretch the legs. Raise the heels and hold the legs parallel to the ground. If you find it hard to take both the legs backwards together, stretch the legs straight one by one and keep them together and stiff. If you try to slightly bend the trunk at the head, the legs would be lifted up of their own accord from the floor. Then it would be easy to stretch the legs backwards. When the posture is correctly assumed, the head, the hips, the thighs, the legs and the feet will be in a straight line parallel to the ground. Practise this asana for five to twenty seconds. Hold the breath at the time of raising the body. This will revitalize the body. Exhale quietly when the asana is completed. One who possesses a sound physique can practise this asana for two to three minutes.

Advantages : (1) This asana gives much exercise in a limited time. It is a great energizing exercise. It amazingly increases the power of digestion.

(2) It cures the diseases caused by the excess of 'vata', 'pitta' and 'kafa' (wind, bile and phlegm). It stops the bleeding caused by piles. It also prevents diabetes.

(3) It strengthens the muscles of the arms, awakens the Kundalini and cures constipation.

(4) It exerts intra-abdominal pressure with the result that the abdominal organs and the lungs become rejuvenated, and it also eliminates the liver disorders.

(5) The practice of this asana stimulates the circulation of the blood in the body. Consequently, the body becomes bright and radiant.

(6) It prevents obesity in the body.

2. VRISHCHIKASANA

'Vrishchika' means a scorpion. In this asana, the body assumes the pose of a scorpion. So it is called Vrishchikasana. Those who can practise Sheershasana or Hastavrikshasana for a long time can practise this asana with ease and comfort.

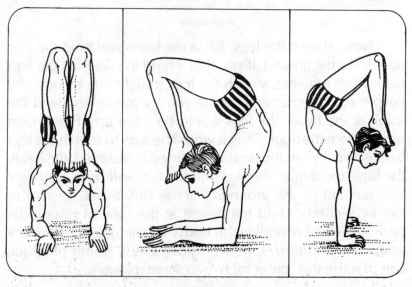

Vrishchikasana

Technique : A beginner should practise this asana with the support of a wall. Place the forearms and the elbows on the floor. Push against the floor lightly with the legs. Slowly move the legs five cms away from the wall and try to balance the body on the forearms. Breathe normally. Practise this for a few days. After achieving proficiency, bend the legs at the knees and try to place the soles on the head. Patient practice will in time impart the necessary ability to balance the body on the palms braced on the ground.

Advantages : (1) This asana strengthens the arms and the shoulders. It gives sufficient exercise to the abdominal muscles.

(2) The spine is turned backward in this asana which brings flexibility and imparts radiance and youth to the body.

(3) It has all the advantages of Sheershasana, Chakrasana and Dhanurasana.

3. BAKASANA

'Baka' means a stork. Bakasana is one among the best of the asanas. Two different techniques have been given here.

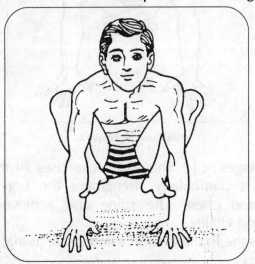

Bakasana (Technique 1)

Technique (Posture 1) : Brace the palms on the floor. Press the shin against the arms. Now, raise the body. Place the toes under the elbows so as to support them. Hold the breath. Hold the position. Gradually, increase the time to the limit of fifteen minutes.

Technique (Posture 2) : Take the position of Bakasana as shown above. In the first type of Bakasana, the soles are supported under the elbows. In the second type, there is a variation. Take the soles backwards and rest them together below the hips as shown in Technique 2. See that the right sole presses against the left sole. The remaining process is the same as shown in the first type.

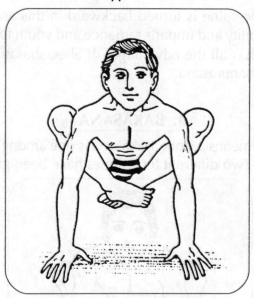

Bakasana (Technique 2)

Advantages : (1) This asana exercises all the parts of the body. It particularly strengthens the organs of the abdomen and chest. The spine also achieves strength, flexibility and vitality.

(2) As the Prana is sublimated in the asana, it bestows mental peace.

(3) It has all the benefits that Utthita Padmasana has.

(4) It stimulates the digestive, the respiratory and the nervous systems.

Note : Kapalabhati performed during this asana bestows many benefits but the exercise should be done after sufficient practice of this asana.

4. TOLASANA

This is a variation of Bakasana. This asana is also called Tulitasana.

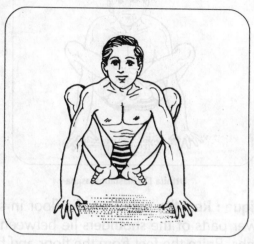

Tolasana

Technique : Practise Bakasana as shown in Bakasana Technique 1. At the last stage of the asana, do not rest the soles under the elbows, but keep them a bit apart in the middle of the arms. This pose is known as Tolasana. Do the remaining part of the exercise as you would do while practising Bakasana. Gradually, increase the time to the limit of fifteen minutes.

Advantages : (1) In the practice of this asana, the eyes are frequently concentrated on the part between the eyebrows. This removes many common defects of the eyes.

(2) This asana has all the benefits of Bakasana.

(3) It cures all the diseases which Utthita Padmasana cures. It has the same benefits as Utthita Padmasana.

5. UTTHITA DWIHASTABHUJASANA

This asana is a variation of Tolasana. It is a little difficult to practise. An aspirant must have strong arms to practise this asana.

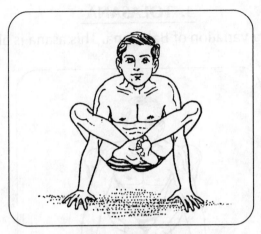

Utthita Dwihastabhujasana

Technique : Rest the palms on the floor in such a way that the lower parts of the shoulders lie between the calves and the thighs. Raise the feet from the floor and balance the entire body on the hands. Interlock the feet. Hold the breath. Slowly increase the duration of time to the limit of five minutes.

Advantages : (1) This asana gives the maximum exercise in the minimum time.

(2) It strengthens the muscles of the arms and the legs.

(3) It cures all the diseases which Utthita Padmasana helps to cure. It has all the benefits of Bakasana.

6. UTTAMANGASANA

To practise Uttamangasana is not so easy as either Lolasana or Kukkutasana. The body should be strong to practise this asana. Gymnasts can perform this asana very easily.

Technique : First sit in the position of Padmasana. Then raise the knees and press them between the chest and the arms. Then raise the body with the force of the arms in such a way that the weight of the body falls on both the arms. While

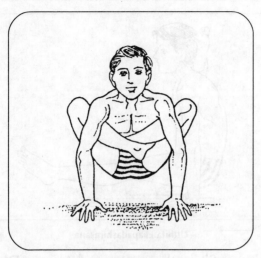

Uttamangasana

raising the body inhale and fill the lungs with air. Hold the breath. Exhale smoothly while coming to the original position. Gradually, increase the time for the practice of this asana. The limit is five minutes.

Advantages : (1) This asana strengthens the joints and the muscles of the arms and the legs.

(2) As it eliminates the weakness of all the abdominal organs and the chest it is more important than Lolasana or Kukkutasana.

(3) The regular practice of this asana roots out diseases like tuberculosis and asthma.

Note : Before an aspirant begins to practise this asana, he is required to acquire physical ability by practising simple and easy asanas.

7. UTTHITA EKAPADASHIRASANA

This asana is comparatively difficult for the beginners. The body should be properly flexible and the arms should be strong for the perfect performance of this asana. Gymnasts can practise this asana with ease and comfort.

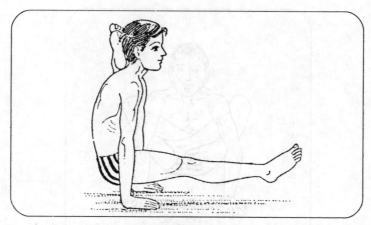

Utthita Ekapadashirasana

Technique : Sit in the posture of Akarna Dhanurasana Technique 2 (See page no. 50). Place the hands on the floor. Raise the entire body with the support of the arms. Keep straight the stretched leg. See that it does not bend at the knees. In the other technique, one has to change the leg. Practise this asana for thirty seconds in the beginning. Gradually, increase the time to three minutes.

Advantages : (1) The wind in the body is sublimated by the practice of this asana. It stimulates gastric fire.

(2) This asana cures constipation.

(3) This asana produces digestive juices in abundance and food is digested well.

(4) It assuages abdominal diseases.

(5) The regular practice of this asana brings delightful peace to the mind and it invigorates the body.

(6) It cures all the diseases cured by Utthita Padmasana.

8. KONASANA

The posture has a shape of an angle formed by the arms and the legs. So it is called Konasana. In this asana, the balance is maintained with the palms and the heels firmly fixed on the ground.

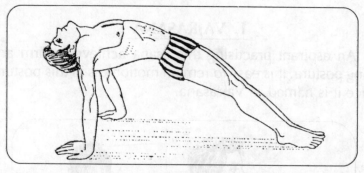

Konasana

Technique : Keep the feet close together. Keep the arms perpendicular to the shoulders and extend the legs. Inhale and with the help of the palms and the heels, raise the trunk upwards. Bend the neck backwards. Keep the arms straight and the chest towards the sky. Hold this position for eight to ten seconds. Then slowly come to the original position. Repeat this asana four to six times.

Advantages : (1) This asana strengthens the shoulders and alleviates the abdominal disorders.

(2) It gives sufficient exercise to the legs and the spine.

(3) This asana is considered to be a variation of Pashchimottanasana. So if it is practised after practising Pashchimottanasana, it gives many benefits.

8. KNEELING POSTURES

1. VAJRASANA

An aspirant practising this asana achieves a firm and strong posture. It is easy to remain motionless in this posture, hence it is named as Vajrasana.

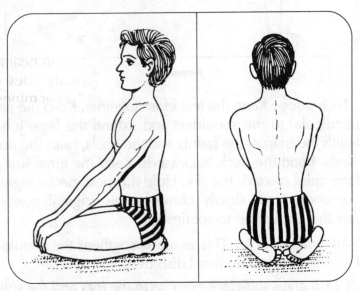

Vajrasana (Side View)   Vajrasana (Rear View)

Technique : Bend the legs at the knees. Place the heels at the sides of the anus in such a way that the thighs rest on the legs and the buttocks rest on the heels. Support the whole body on the knees and the ankles. Breathe normally while performing this asana. The knees and the ankles will perhaps ache in the beginning but this ache or pain will disappear by itself. Stretch the arms and place the hands on the knees. Keep the knees close by. Sit erect keeping the trunk, the neck and the head in a straight line. This is a very simple posture and one can hold this posture with ease for a longer time.

Advantages : (1) This asana helps digestion and eliminates gas-trouble.

(2) The constant and systematic practice of this asana alleviates the pain of the knees, the legs, the feet and the thighs.

(3) Vajrasana energises Kandasthana situated about thirty cms away from the anus. This Kandasthana is considered to be the centre of 72,000 nadis (tubular channels).

(4) The regular practice of this asana increases the secretion from the glands. It also increases the white blood corpuscles produced in the spleen, the tonsils, the marrow and in other parts of the body. This is beneficial to health.

(5) One who practises this asana regularly does not suffer from fever, constipation, indigestion and other minor or major ailments.

Note : This is the only asana, which, if practised immediately after meals, stimulates digestion.

2. SUPTA VAJRASANA

Supta Vajrasana is similar to Ardha Shavasana. It can be placed in the category of Matsyasana. One should practise it only after one masters Vajrasana. Compared to Vajrasana, Supta Vajrasana requires more strength and flexibility of the spine.

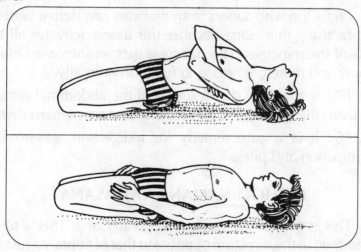

Supta Vajrasana (Techniques 1-2)

Technique : Attain Vajrasana. Then with the support of the elbows lie with the back on the ground. The back should touch the ground. Interlace the arms and put them on the chest. Tilt the head as far back as possible. Hold this position for eight to ten seconds. In the beginning, the back may not wholly touch the ground. The lower part of the back may remain in a raised position. A few days' practice will enable one to practise this asana correctly. This asana can be practised three or four times a day.

Advantages : (1) This asana helps to remove certain defects of the spine. As the spine is arched backwards in this asana, it removes a hunch, if any. The spine becomes flexible and elastic.

(2) The regular practice of this asana awakens and sublimates Kundalini Shakti.

(3) This asana exercises and activates the thorax, the spine and the neck.

(4) It stimulates the secretion from all the glands and makes the glands active with the result that one feels healthy and joyful.

(5) It strengthens the joints and the muscles of the legs.

(6) One who suffers from diabetes can derive benefits by practising this asana because this asana activates all the cells of the pancreas. The pancreas gets an increased blood supply and therefore begins to function normally.

(7) It alleviates the disorders of the abdominal organs, the liver, the kidney, the spleen, etc. and strengthens them.

(8) It is a sure remedy for indigestion, gas-trouble, constipation and piles.

3. BHOO-NAMANA-VAJRASANA

This is one of the variations of Vajrasana. This is to be performed in the direction opposite to that of Supta Vajrasana. Some consider this asana to be one kind of Yoga-Mudra.

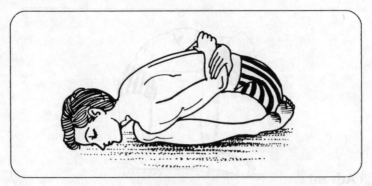

Bhoo-Namana-Vajrasana

Technique : Attain Vajrasana. Slowly and cautiously bend the trunk forward. Take the arms to the back. Hold the right forearm with the left hand and the left forearm with the right hand. Fill the air in the lungs. Slowly exhale and stretch the neck downward so that the nose touches the ground. Gradually, increase the time to the limit of ten seconds.

Advantages : (1) This asana eliminates the weakness of the intestines and the stomach. It also removes disorders of the liver and the laxity of the pancreas.

(2) It increases the elasticity of the spine and also strengthens the muscles of the abdomen and the chest.

(3) It cures constipation.

(4) It cures diseases such as diabetes, abdominal disorders, cold, gas-trouble, loss of appetite, nocturnal discharge, insomnia, asthma, dysentery and indigestion.

(5) It stimulates gastric fire.

4. USHTRASANA

This asana belongs to the category of Vajrasana. It should be practised after practising Vajrasana. 'Ushtra' means a camel. In this asana almost all the limbs of the body are arched like those of a camel. So it is called Ushtrasana.

Technique : Kneel on the ground as in Vajrasana keeping the distance of about fifteen cms between the knees and between the heels. Breathe deeply. Hold the right ankles

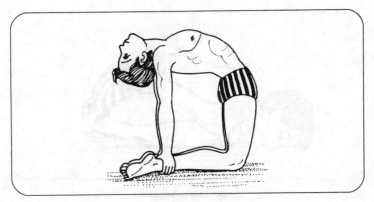

Ushtrasana

firmly with the right hand and the left ankles with the left hand. Raise the arms and take them behind the neck. Breathe in the normal way. Hold this position for six to eight seconds. Repeat this asana two or three times a day.

Advantages : (1) This asana activates the respiratory system and so it is beneficial to those who suffer from asthma.

(2) The body becomes weak when there are impurities in the blood or when the flesh and the semen are diseased. In such cases, this asana is beneficial.

(3) This asana cures diseases caused by 'vata', 'pitta' and 'kafa' (wind, bile and phlegm).

(4) The practice of this asana cures all types of diseases related to fistula. It has a soothing effect on menorrhagia and diabetes.

(5) It removes pain in the neck, the shoulders and the spine.

(6) It improves eyesight.

(7) It helps to alleviate headache and trouble in the voice and the tonsils.

(8) It gives proper exercise to the chest and makes it shapely.

5. VRUSHASANA

'Vrusha' means a bull. An aspirant who performs this asana resembles the image of manliness. He is believed to be a 'man-bull' and so this asana is called Vrushasana. Physical flaccidity in a young body is a sign of old age. It indicates physical weakness. This asana helps to preserve youth.

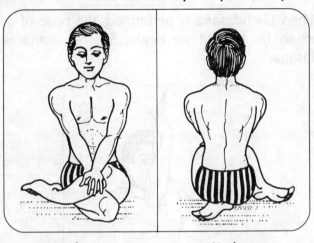

Vrushasana
(Front View)

Vrushasana
(Rear View)

Technique : Bend the right leg at the knee and place the heel under the anus. Place the left knee on the right knee in such a way that the left heel touches the right thigh. Sit erect and place the palm of the right hand on the knee. Then place the palm of the left hand on it. Breathe in the normal way. Direct your sight and attention to the navel.

Advantages : (1) It stimulates blood-circulation making the body energetic and the mind peaceful.

(2) It makes the respiratory system function in a proper order.

(3) It cures diseases such as waste of semen, gas-trouble, nocturnal discharges, indigestion, lumbago, insomnia, cardiac trouble, asthma and dysentery.

(4) It awakens Kundalini Shakti which enters the mouth of the Sushumna.

(5) It strengthens all the muscles of the body.

9. LEG-POSTURES

(Standing Postures)

1. GARUDASANA

When Garudasana is performed, the pose of the body appears to be that of an eagle. So this asana is called Garudasana.

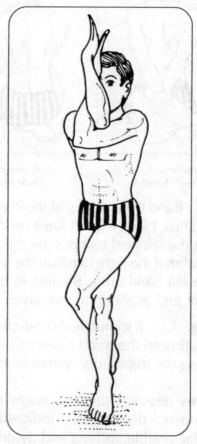

Garudasana

Technique : Stand erect. Keep the right leg straight on the ground and bring the left leg over the right thigh above the right knee. The left leg should be entwined around the right leg in the same way as a creeper encircles the trunk of a tree and sticks to it. The left thigh should be entwined around the right thigh. Interlock the arms in the same manner. The palms should touch each other. Arrange the fingers in such way that they look like the beak of an eagle. Keep the arms in front of the face. Breathe in the normal way. Hold this position for eight to ten seconds. Change the hands and the legs alternately.

Advantages : (1) This asana strengthens the legs. One can balance the body on one leg.

(2) In this asana, the blood vessels are stretched. So they become strong.

(3) It removes the swelling of cells of the testicles.

(4) It cures rheumatism of the arms and the legs.

(5) It alleviates pain in the thighs and the calf muscles.

(6) This asana is helpful for restraining the mind.

2. VRUKSHASANA

'Vruksha' means a tree. In this asana, the body assumes the shape of a tree. So it is called Vrukshasana.

Technique : Stand on either leg. If difficulty is experienced to balance the body on one leg, take the support of a wall. Bend the other leg at the knee and place its heel at the root of the thigh of the former leg as shown in the figure. Join the palms and raise the arms straight over the head as if you are making an obeisance to the sky. Straighten the elbows. Inhale slowly. Hold this position for about ten seconds. Then repeat the pose, standing on the other leg. This exercise can be practised four to six times a day.

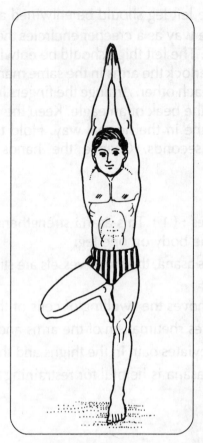

Vrukshasana

Advantages : (1) The pose tones up all the joints of the body.

(2) It supplies blood to the blood vessels of the toes, the knees, the elbows, etc. in sufficient quantity.

(3) The hands and the legs become flexible by the practice of this asana. It makes the chest shapely.

3. VATAYANASANA

In this asana,the body remains in a half standing position with the support of the heel of one leg and the knee of the second leg. The body assumes the pose worshipping God.

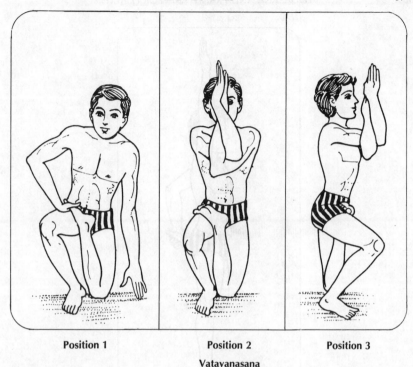

| Position 1 | Position 2 | Position 3 |

Vatayanasana

Technique : Stand erect. Hold the left leg and place the heel on the thigh or at the root of the genitals. Let the left knee slowly touch the ground. Keep the position of the arms as shown in the figure (Position 1). Then as in Garudasana entwine the hands and assume 'Namaskara-Mudra' as shown in the figure (Positions 2 and 3). Look straight. Inhale slowly. Take the position in which the knee of the bent leg touches the right heel. Then slowly come to standing position and repeat the exercise with the second leg.

Advantages : (1) This asana strengthens the legs. It removes the pain in the ankles and the knee-joints.

(2) This asana can be practised for praying to God.

4. SANTULANASANA

In this asana, one has to balance the body on one leg, hence it is called Santulanasana.

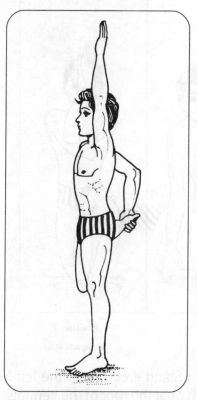

Santulanasana

Technique : Stand straight and erect on the ground. Keep the body straight and erect. Look straight. Keep the arms on the sides. Bend either leg at the knee, keeping the knee facing downwards and the heel upwards. Hold the foot of this leg with the corresponding hand. Raise the other arm close to the ear. Hold this position for eight to ten seconds. Repeat this exercise with the other leg. In the beginning, practise this asana four times a day. Later, it can be practised six times a day.

Advantages : (1) This asana exercises every joint of the body.

(2) It alleviates the pain in the joints.

(3) It properly exercises the ankles, the knees and the fingers. This exercise teaches one how to maintain balance on one leg.

5. NATARAJASANA

The posture of the body while practising this asana resembles Nataraja. So this asana is called Natarajasana. The pose inspires one to go ahead and work.

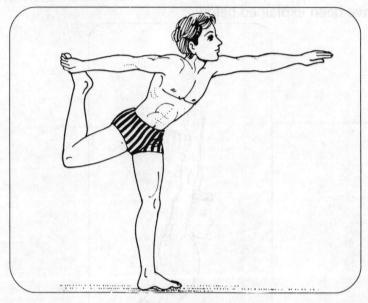

Natarajasana

Technique : Stand erect with both the legs straight. Keep the arms straight by the sides and look straight. Bend either leg at the knee and raise it backwards. Hold the foot with the corresponding hand. Stretch the other arm in the opposite direction and look straight in that direction. Hold the position for eight to ten seconds. Repeat the exercise standing on the other leg. In the beginning, this asana can be practised four times a day. Later, it can be practised six times a day.

Advantages : (1) This asana exercises all the joints of the body.

(2) It gives sufficient exercise to the shoulders, the hips, the knees, the ankles, the palms, the fingers and the spine.

(3) It relieves the pain in the waist and makes the waist flexible.

6. UTKATASANA

Utkatasana is considered to be one of the best asanas. It strengthens the toes and the joints and the muscles of the feet. There are two ways to perform this asana. Both the techniques have been explained below.

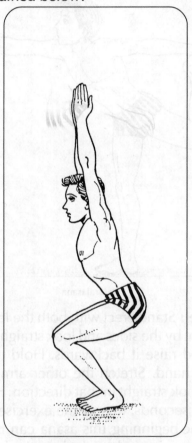

Utkatasana (Technique 1)

Technique 1 : Stand with the legs together. Raise the body on the heels and bring the arms straight over the head and join the palms. Then slowly lower the trunk. This asana does not require much strength to practise it. An aspirant should only know how to balance the body. One who is slim but has a strong physique can practise this asana with ease and comfort.

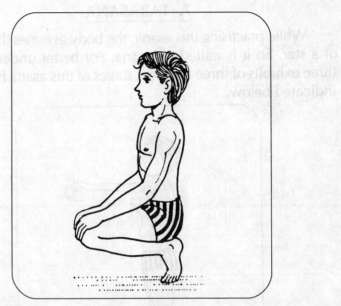

Utkatasana (Technique 2)

Technique 2 : Stand with the arms by the sides. Lift the body five to seven cms above the floor and balance it on the toes. Slowly lower the trunk and sit on the soles. The body will balance on the front part of the feet. The hips will touch the heels. Hold this position for eight to ten seconds. This asana is very useful in the practice known as 'Bastikriya'. Slowly increase the duration of the practice of this asana. The limit is three minutes.

Advantages : (1) This asana strengthens the muscles of the wrists and the feet.

(2) It is beneficial to those who suffer from elephantiasis.

(3) It gives sufficient exercise to all the joints and the muscles of the legs.

(4) It closes the exits of the 'Ida' and the 'Pingala' nadis and lifeforce (energy) begins to flow into the 'Sushumna'.

(5) The regular practice of this asana awakens Kundalini Shakti.

(6) It cures fistula, dropsy, constipation, abdominal disease, impurification of blood, skin disease, flatulence, heart-trouble, arthritis and other diseases.

7. TARASANA

While practising this asana, the body assumes the posture of a star. So it is called Tarasana. For better understanding, three exhibits of three different stages of this asana have been indicated below.

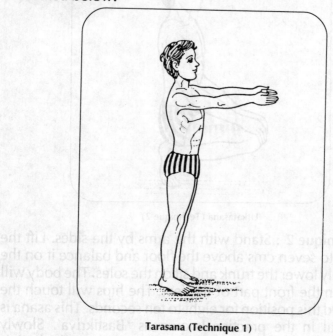

Tarasana (Technique 1)

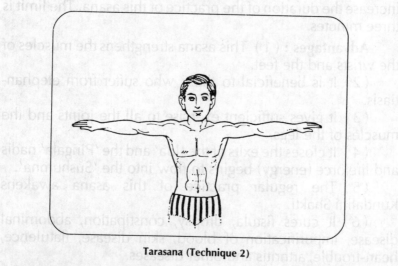

Tarasana (Technique 2)

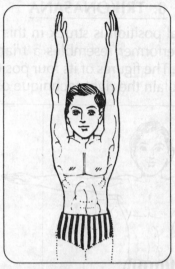

Tarasana (Technique 3)

Technique : Stand straight making an angle of 45° between the feet. Keep the arms in front of you. Keep the palms facing each other and stretch the arms in the line with the shoulders. (See Technique 1.) Then keep the palms downwards facing the ground and stretch the arms on the sides in the line with the shoulders as shown in Technique 2. Then bring the arms upwards and keep the palms facing each other. (See Technique 3.) Hold the position for two seconds at each stage. After completing the third stage, bring the body to its original position. Repeat this asana three to four times. With repeated practice, this asana can be practised six times daily.

Advantages : (1) This asana strengthens the lungs and the chest. It is very much beneficial to those who suffer from asthma.

(2) It activates the respiratory system.

(3) It expands the chest and makes it shapely (symmetrical).

(4) The regular practice of this asana helps to increase the height of the body to some extent.

8. TRIKONASANA

When the final position is struck in this Yogic exercise, the body of the performer resembles a triangle, hence the name Trikonasana. The figures of its four positions have been given below to explain the right technique of this asana.

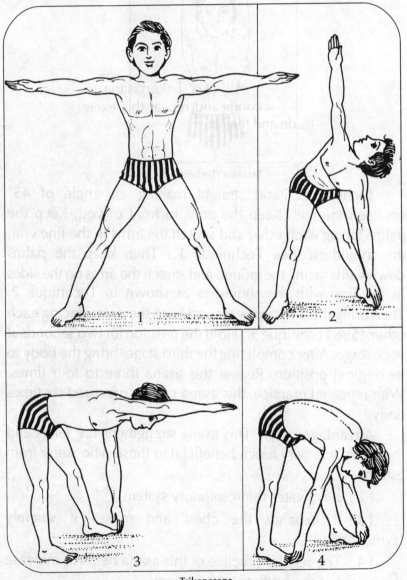

Trikonasana

Technique : Stand erect keeping a distance of about 75 cms between the feet. Stretch the arms sideways. Then raise them to the level of the shoulders. Let the palms face the ground. Stand erect. (See figure 1.) Then bend the trunk to the left side and touch the left toes with the left hand. Stretch the right arm upwards and straighten it. Keep the eyes fixed on the right arm. Bring the left hand near the left toe. (See figure 2.) Keep the left hand in the same position and rotate the right arm from over the waist and bring it to the head level. Look downward. (See figure 3.) Then touch the right toes with the right hand. This is the final position of Trikonasana. (See figure 4.) Rest for five to ten seconds and repeat this exercise with the right arm downside and the left arm upside. Hold each position for two seconds. Practise this asana four or five times a day.

Advantages : (1) This asana relieves the stiffness of the neck.

(2) It relieves the pain in the joints of the neck and the shoulders. It also exercises the spinal cord, the hips, the thighs, the arms and the fingers.

(3) It makes the spine flexible and develops the mental power. This asana is also beneficial to the eyes.

9. PADAHASTASANA

If 'Pashchimottanasana' is attained in a standing posture, it becomes a different yogic exercise known as 'Padahastasana'. This asana is also called 'Sthita Pashchi mottanasana'. Some people call it 'Hastapada Mangasana'.

Technique : Stand erect. Keep the arms by the sides. Keep the heels close together. Keep some gap between the feet. Raise both the arms. Slowly bend forward at the waist. Keep the knees stiff and firm. The legs should not bend at the knees. Also do not let the arms bend at the elbows. Keep the palms under the feet as shown in the figure. Slowly exhale while bending low and contract the stomach. Now put your forehead between the knees. If it is difficult to bend low

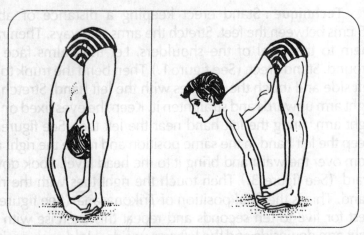

Padahastasana

because of fat around the abdomen, try to bend the body slowly; do not bend the knees. Hold this position for two to ten seconds.

Advantages : (1) This asana removes the superfluous fat from the body making the body light.

(2) It directs the 'apanvayu' downwards and out at the anus.

(3) It has all the benefits of Pashchimottanasana.

(4) It rectifies any unevenness in length in the leg owing to the fracture of any bones either in the leg or the thigh.

10. CHAKRASANA

In practising this asana, the spine is twisted in such a way that the body forms a semicircular shape, hence this asana is called 'Chakrasana'. It resembles a rainbow.

Technique : Lie flat on the back. Draw the legs in till the heels are close to the hips and the soles touch the ground. The gap between the legs should be of four to six inches. Bend the arms at the elbows and place them on the ground on either side of the head.

Raise the body from the waist to the hind part of the head as shown in the figures 2 and 3 and breathe in the normal way. Tilt the head backwards as far as possible. Keep the hands straight. Keep the body steady. Do not shift either the arms or the legs from their positions. Raise the back as far

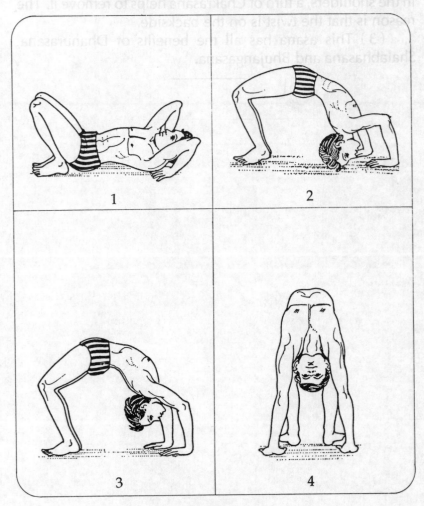

Chakrasana

as it allows it to do. (See figure 4.) Remain in this position for about a minute. Then inhale and lower the body to the ground and bring it to the original position. Then breathe normally.

Advantages : (1) Through this asana, an aspirant can make his spine quite elastic. Elasticity of the spine preserves youth for a very long time.

(2) This asana is an adjunct to Sarvangasana. When a long turn of Sarvangasana gives one a cramped neck or pain in the shoulders, a turn of Chakrasana helps to remove it. The reason is that the twist is on the backside.

(3) This asana has all the benefits of Dhanurasana, Shalabhasana and Bhujangasana.

10. HEAD-POSTURES

1. SHEERSHASANA

'Sheersha' means a head. This asana is the head-stand pose. This asana is called the king of asanas. It is also known as 'Kapaliasana', 'Vrukshasana' and 'Viparitakarani'. Four stages in figures (preparation) have been given below for the better guidance to an aspirant to practise this asana with ease.

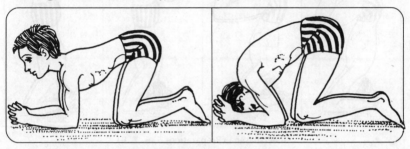

Sheershasana (Preparations 1, 2)

Technique : The first stage : Spread a blanket four-fold or cloth on the floor and kneel on it. Interlock the fingers of the hands and put them on the floor.

The second stage : Now place the top of the head on the clasped hands between the elbows. Raise the legs slowly. In the beginning, keep the legs raised for five to fifteen seconds. Increase fifteen seconds every week. Later, practise this asana for half an hour.

Practise keeping the legs raised as shown in the figure. Do

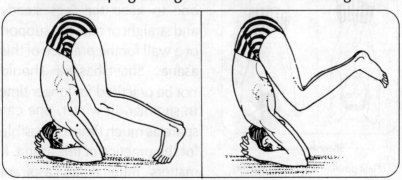

Sheershasana (Preparations 3, 4)

109

the exercise patiently with caution. Keep the heels of the legs upwards in the direction of the sky. Breathe in the normal way. Then slowly lower the legs.

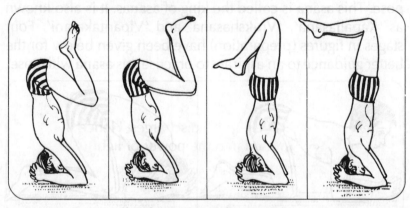

Sheershasana (Preparations 5, 6, 7, 8)

Sheershasana should be practised only on an empty stomach. If time permits, perform Sheershasana twice a day,

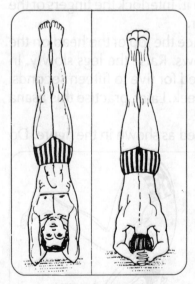

Sheershasana

(Final position and backside pose)

morning and evening. Practise it very slowly without jerks. While standing on the head, breathe slowly. Breathe through the nose and never through the mouth. A beginner should take the help of someone to keep the legs steady and straight or take the support of a wall for the practice of this asana. Sheershasana should not be practised for longer time in summer. In winter, one can spare as much time as possible for the practice of this asana. It matters little if an aspirant keeps his eyes open or closed while practising this asana. But if the duration for the practice of this asana is long, it is better to keep the eyes closed. This will enable one to meditate. After the completion of this asana, relax for five minutes. One should necessarily take a cup of milk or light snacks after taking complete rest.

Note : Sheershasana should invariably be followed by Shavasana for rest.

Advantages : (1) This asana helps an aspirant to observe celibacy. It preserves energy and gives vitality. It adds to his vigour.

(2) It prevents nocturnal discharges. Hence the power of semen is transformed into the power of light *(Ojas).*

(3) As this asana reverses the normal effects of gravity, it encourages an abundant influx of arterial blood to the brain.

(4) It adds to the mental power, improves memory and awakens Kundalini Shakti.

(5) This asana is a panacea (cure-all) for all diseases. It stimulates digestive juices and kindles gastric fire. Also, it cures the diseases of the eyes, the nose, the head and the throat. It also cures diseases like diabetes and asthma.

(6) Yoga Tatva Upanishad says, "He who practises the headstand (Sheershasana) for three hours every day conquers time." Sheershasana, indeed, is a nectar.

* Caution : On reading about the benefits acquired by the practice of Sheershasana, one should not be too zealous to practise it beyond one's capacity. Headstand asanas should not be done by those who have ear or throat infections, insomnia or weak eyes.

2. URDHVA PADMASANA

In this asana, Padmasana is done with the headstand (Sheershasana). There are two techniques for the performance of this asana.

They are explained below :

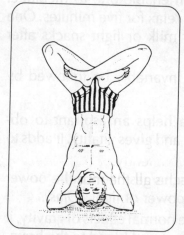

Urdhva
Padmasana (Technique 1)

Technique 1 : First attain the posture of Sheershasana. Slowly bend the right leg and place it on the left thigh. Then place the left leg on the right thigh. Do this exercise slowly and very carefully. Those who are able to stay in the position of Sheershasana for ten to fifteen minutes should only try to perform this asana, otherwise there is a possibility of falling down.

Technique 2 : Keep the head on the ground. Place the palms on the ground one on each side of the head at some distance from the head. Raise the body keeping the balance on the hands. Attain Padmasana and bring the crossed legs vertically in line with the head.

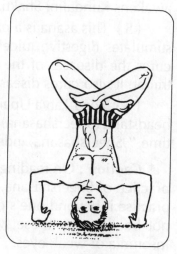

Urdhva
Padmasana (Technique 2)

Initially, this asana should be practised with the support of a wall. Some physical strength is required for the practice of this asana. One who can balance the body on the ground without any support can perform this asana smoothly. Inhale through the nose while practising this asana and never inhale through the mouth. Practise this asana for five to ten minutes at the start. Increase the time gradually.

Note : The practice of this asana should be preceded by Pranayama.

Advantages : (1) This asana has all the advantages of Sheershasana and Padmasana. One who practises this asana achieves the perfect control of the body.

(2) It strengthens the brain by supplying it with an abundant flow of blood. This in turn increases the power of meditation and sharpens the intellect.

(3) It improves the eyesight and removes the weakness of the ears, the chest, the heart and other organs.

(4) It supplies arterial blood to all the internal glands with the result that they function efficiently.

(5) It strengthens and nourishes all the muscles, bones and sense organs.

3. URDHVA SAMYUKTA PADMASANA

This is a very useful asana. Proficiency is accomplished after some vigorous efforts. There are two techniques for the performance of this asana. Both the techniques are explained below.

Technique 1 : First attain Sheershasana. Then fold the legs double at the knees so that the legs are perpendicular to the torso. The practice of this asana needs some strength and vigour.

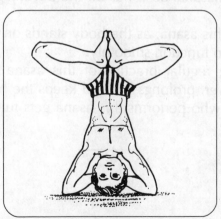

Urdhava Samyukta Padmasana (Technique 1)

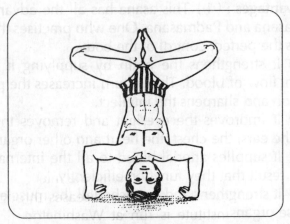

Urdhva Samyukta Padmasana (Technique 2)

Technique 2 : Keep the head on the ground. Place the palms at some distance from the head firmly fixed on the ground. Then raise the body with the force of the hands, and fold the legs double at the knees. Join the heels. It is advisable to take the support of a wall in the initial stage. Only those who can practise Sheershasana for ten to fifteen minutes should try to practise this asana. Initially, practise this asana for five minutes. Later, slowly increase the time up to the limit of fifteen minutes.

Advantages : (1) This asana belongs to the category of Urdhva Padmasana. So it has all the advantages of Urdhva Padmasana.

(2) In this asana, as the body stands on the head, the veins begin to function smoothly.

(3) The regular practice of this asana increases the memory power, prolongs life and keeps the body in sound health. One who performs this asana gets full control over the body.

11. YOGIC EXERCISES AND THE CURE OF DISEASES – AN INDEX

From times immemorial the Indian method of Yogic exercises has been known and practised. Yoga has been practised for thousands of years for keeping the human body free from diseases. Yoga, in fact, is a scientific system of physiotherapy. Today, Yoga is practised not only in order to keep the body free from diseases but also as a remedy for diseases. Recently, several institutes in the international field have been established to diagnose diseases through Yoga. One such Yoga institute is run at Washington (D. C.) in the U. S. A. In India, too, several such institutes have been established : (1) Kaivalyadham, Lonavala, Pune, (Maharashtra); (2) Yoga Institute, Santa Cruz, Bombay; (3) Yoga For Life and Living, Vishvayatana Yogashram, Delhi; (4) Bharatiya Yoga Sansthan, Patna, Bihar and several others. At Lonavala, extensive research work on Yoga is being carried out. Today, many incurable and long-standing diseases can be cured through Yoga.

The Yoga treatment is perfectly scientific. It is an auto-treatment method. Yoga therapy includes nutritious food, restraint and a code of conduct to be followed by the diseased. The treatment for diseases through Yoga is itself a vast and deep study. It is not possible to do full justice to the subject in this small book. The book, therefore, includes only the common beneficial effects of Yogasanas on various diseases. Those who desire to get detailed information should seek for the advice of Yoga institutes mentioned above and their experts. The detailed information regarding asanas has been mentioned elsewhere in this book. With the help of and guidance from information that, an aspirant should start practising asanas.

Diseases	Yogasanas
1. TB. and asthma	Siddhasana, Sheershasana, Sarvangasana, Matsyasana, Ardha Matsyendrasana, Supta Vajrasana and Bhujangasana.
2. Diabetes	Siddhasana, Sheershasana, Sarvangasana, Matsyasana, Ardha Matsyendrasana, Halasana, Chakrasana and Mayurasana.
3. Sex-sublimation, pyorrhoea and colic	Siddhasana, Sheershasana, Sarvangasana, Matsyasana, Ardha Matsyendrasana, Padmasana, Vajrasana and Pashchimottanasana.
4. Pain in the ears, eyes, and nose	Siddhasana, Sarvangasana, Matsyasana and Ardha Matsyendrasana.
5. Loss of menstruation, painful menstruation, menorrhagia and the diseases related to the uterus and ovary	Sarvangasana, Shalabhasana, Pashchimottanasana and Bhujangasana. (These asanas should not be practised during pregnancy.)
6. Chronic bronchitis, cough, difficulty in breathing	Matsyasana and Shalabhasana.
7. Disorders of the digestive system	Sarvangasana, Vajrasana, Pashchimottanasana and Baddha Padmasana.
8. Enlargement of the liver and the spleen	Sarvangasana, Halasana, Mayurasana and Baddha Padmasana.
9. Chronic constipation	Halasana, Mayurasana, Dhanurasana, Matsyasana and Padahastasana.
10. Hernia, Elephantiasis, shortness of a leg or of an arm	Garudasana, Trikonasana and Utkatasana.
11. Piles	Siddhasana, Pashchimottanasana, Sheershasana, Gomukhasana and Mahamudra.

Diseases	Yogasanas
12. Dysentery	Baddha Padmasana and Kukkutasana.
13. Rheumatism in the joints	Vrushchikasana, Sheershasana, Pashchimottanasana and Sarvangasana.
14. Leucoderma	Sheershasana, Padmasana, Siddhasana, Simhasana, Gomukhasana, Vakrasana and Vrukshasana.
15. Fatness (Obesity)	Mandukasana, Pashchimottanasana, Mayurasana, Supta Vajrasana, Dhanurasana and Ardha Matsyendrasana.
16. High blood pressure	Vajrasana, Siddhasana, Padmasana, Matsyasana and Shavasana
17. Low blood pressure	Sarvangasana, Halasana, Vajrasana, Padmasana, Siddhasana and Pashchimottanasana.
18. Throat-trouble	Matsyasana, Simhasana, Supta Vajrasana and Sarvangasana.
19. Headache	Pashchimottanasana, Halasana, Sarvangasana and Shavasana.
20. Hernia	Matsyasana, Sarvangasana and Suptavajrasana.
21. Heart-disease (Cardiac trouble)	Shavasana, Baddha Padmasana and Siddhasana.
22. Insomnia	Sarvangasana, Shavasana and Surya Namaskara
23. Menstrual troubles	Dhanurasana, Matsyasana, Supta Vajrasana and Pashchimottanasana.
24. Drowsiness	Lolasana, Kukkutasana, Uttamangasana, Bakasana, Tolasana, Utthita Dwihastabhujasana and Utthita Ekapadashirasana.
25. Intestinal diseases	Lolasana, Garbhasana, Baddhahasta Padmasana and Surya Namaskara.
26. Lumbar pain	Vakrasana, Tolangulasana, Halasana and Surya Namaskara.

Diseases	Yogasanas
27. Dermatic diseases	Padmasana, Siddhasana, Simhasana, Veerasana, Utkatasana, Mandukasana, Supta Vrajasana and Vrukshasana.
28. Diseases related to the chest and the lungs	Baddha Padmasana, Utkatasana, Sarvangasana, Viparitakarani Mudra, Sheershasana, Vrukshasana and Surya Namaskara.
29. Fever, chronic fever	Garbhasana, Utthita Padmasana, Siddhasana, Gomukhasana and Shavasana.
30. Impotence	Padmasana, Siddhasana, Simhasana, Mandukasana, Vajrasana, Supta Vajrasana and Gomukhasana.
31. Impurities of veins	Lolasana and Utthita Ekapadashirasana
32. Leg-ailments	Baddha Padmasana, Utkatasana, Akarna Dhanurasana, Tolangulasana and Padmasana.
33. Kidney stone	Matsyendrasana, Matsyasana, Tolangulasana and Vajrasana.
34. Paralysis	Padmasana, Veerasana, Parvatasana, Matsyendrasana, Matsyasana, Siddhasana, Simhasana and Mandukasana.
35. Derangement of bile	Halasana, Vartulasana and Shalabhasana.
36. Morbid excitement, hysteria	Padmasana, Vakrasana, Ardha Matsyendrasana, Vrushasana, Mandukasana and Vajrasana.
37. Leprosy	Padmasana, Matsyendrasana, Siddhasana, Simhasana, Gomukhasana and Veerasana.
38. Blood impurities, Loss of blood	Lolasana, Kukkutasana, Bakasana, Utkatasana, Sarvangasana, Sheershasana and Vrukshasana.
39. Elephantiasis	Matsyendrasana, Utkatasana, Utthita Ekapadashirasana.

12. SURYA NAMASKARA

Surya Namaskara signifies paying homage to (Lord) Sun deity. It is a very ancient Indian system of exercise. Facing east, in the early hours of morning, one standing with serene mind offers prayer to Lord Surya with Surya Namaskara. Along with physical drill, Surya Namaskara has religious importance also.

Surya Namaskara is a graceful combined sequence of twelve positions. Through this sequence of twelve positions, the whole body is well exercised. Surya Namaskara also improves eye lustre. As a matter of fact, these twelve positions are ten different asanas, as well as two positions : the initial position and the final position. As all these exercises are simple, every one can do them easily. These twelve positions make one complete Surya Namaskara and twenty-five such Surya Namaskaras make one round.

Surya Namaskara should be practised always in an open and clean place. Do not attempt Surya Namaskara when you begin to breathe hard. Practise Surya Namaskara on one leg changing the leg alternately.

Below you will find the twelve positions of Surya Namaskara fully explained and illustrated. Each position has been shown with the name of the asana. The advantages of each position have been fully explained. Thus, all care has been taken to enable an aspirant with proper understanding to practise it easily.

While practising Surya Namaskara, recite the following prayer. Then recite the different names of the Sun god at each position and offer him mental obeisance.

Prayer

ध्येय: सदा सवितृमण्डलमध्यवर्ती
नारायण: सरसिजासनसन्निविष्ट: ।
केयूरवान् मकरकुण्डलवान् किरीटी
हारी हिरण्मयवपुर्धृतशङ्खचक्र: ।।

Names to be recited at each respective position :

(१) ॐ मित्राय नम: । (२) ॐ रवये नम: । (३) ॐ सूर्याय नम: ।
(४) ॐ भानवे नम: । (५) ॐ खगाय नम: । (६) ॐ पूष्णे नम: ।
(७) ॐ हिरण्यगर्भाय नम: । (८) ॐ मरीचये नम: । (९) ॐ आदित्याय नम: ।
(१०) ॐ सवित्रे नम: । (११) ॐ अर्काय नम: । (१२) ॐ भास्कराय नम: ।

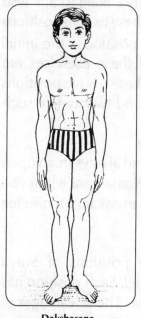

Dakshasana

1. DAKSHASANA

Technique : In the first position of Surya Namaskara, meditate on the Sun god and feel oneness with all the creatures of the world. Then keep the head, the neck and the whole body erect. Keep the knees close together, shoulders straight and the hands downwards at the sides of the body. Stand erect with the chest expanded. Direct the eyes to the tip of the nose. 'Daksha' means to stand in attention. So the first position is called Dakshasana.

Advantages : (1) It cures skin diseases and the ailments of the waist. It strengthens the back and rejuvenates the legs.

(2) As the eyes are fixed on the tip of the nose, the mind is restrained.

(3) The countenance becomes bright and radiant.

(4) For students, it is a very easy method to obtain health and assert personality.

(5) Concentrated meditation increases self-confidence.

2. NAMASKARASANA

Technique : Keep your folded hands in the posture of Namaskara touching the chest. Push the chest out. Pull the stomach inwards. Fill the lungs with air. Look straight, the body, the head and the neck to remain in a vertical straight line. Close the mouth. Inhale and hold the breath.

Advantages : It cures throat-troubles, improves the voice and gives pace to the mind.

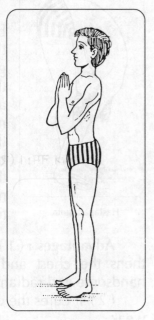

Namaskarasana

3. PARVATASANA

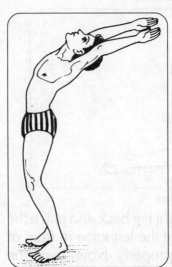

Technique : Stretch the arms up and arch the body backwards from the waist, the eyes to remain open and look at the sky. Bend backwards as far as possible. Expand the chest and push it forwards.

Advantages : It nourishes the shoulders and the alimentary canal. It cures the diseases of the alimentary canal. It improves the eyesight.

Parvatasana

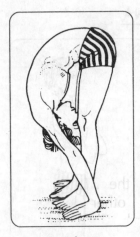

Hastapadasana

4. HASTAPADASANA

Technique : Continue holding the breath and bend down without bending the knees. Press the palms down on the ground, and the fingertips in line with the toes. The fingertips should touch one another. Then touch the knees with the nose or the forehead without bending the knees and exhale. Exhaling should be through the nose only, never through the mouth. In the early stages, the fingers may not touch the ground but the position will be attained after some practice.

Advantages : (1) It cures abdominal diseases, strengthens the chest and the hands and the body becomes handsome and radiant.

(2) It cures the diseases of the toes and invigorates the weak.

5. EKAPADAPRASARANASANA

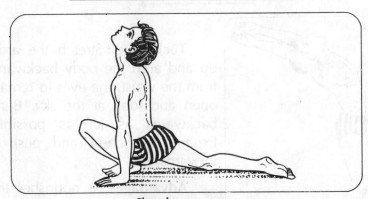

Ekapadaprasaranasana

Technique : Inhale. Take the right leg back and place the knee and the toes on the floor. Bring the left knee in front of the left armpit. Press the abdomen properly. Now, bend the neck as far backwards as possible throwing the chest out. Look up and hold the breath.

Advantages : (1) This position gives pressure to the small intestines and pulls the vessels carrying semen. Hence it cures the diseases of the liver and constipation.

(2) This exercise is beneficial to those who have lost their virility.

(3) It cures the diseases of the throat such as tonsillitis.

6. BHUDHARASANA

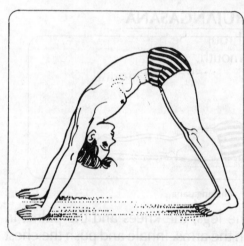

Bhudharasana

Technique : Retaining the breath, move the other leg backwards. Place the toes, the ankles and the knees in such a way that they touch one another. Keep the head, the waist and the elbows in a straight line. Support the weight of the body on the hands and the toes.

Advantages : (1) It cures the ailments of the hands, the legs and particularly the knees. It reduces fat around the waist. This position is a sure remedy for abdominal disorders.

7. ASHTANGAPRANIPATASANA

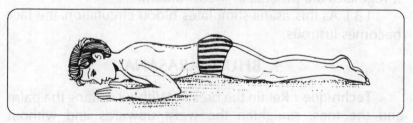

Ashtangapranipatasana

Technique : Retaining the breath, place the knees on the floor. Lower the chest so that it touches the ground. Let the chin touch the lower part of the throat. Lower the forehead so that it touches the ground without allowing the nose to touch the ground. Pull the stomach inwards. See that it does not touch the ground. Then exhale. The chest should lie between the arms.

Advantages : (1) This asana strengthens the arms.

(2) If women practise this asana before pregnancy, infants feeding on breast are saved from various diseases.

8. BHUJANGASANA

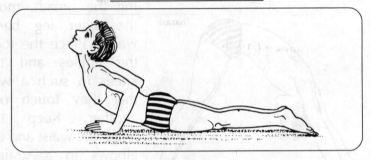

Bhujangasana

Technique : Keep the legs, the knees and the palms in the same position. Stretch the arms. Inhale and push the chest forward. Bend the waist backwards and bend the neck as far back as possible. Look up and hold the breath.

Advantages : (1) This asana removes paleness of the body and makes it ruddy.

(2) It cures the diseases related to the ovary or testicles. It regulates the process of menstruation.

(3) As this asana stimulates blood circulation, the face becomes lustrous.

9. BHUDHARASANA

Technique : Retain the breath. Without shifting the palm and the toes, straighten the waist upwards and without bending the knees stretch the body back. Let the chin touch the chest. Pull the stomach inwards. Stretch the thighs upwards. Rest the heels completely on the floor.

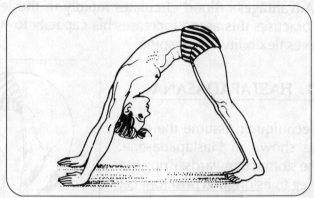

Bhudharasana

Advantages : (1) It prevents rheumatism, paralysis and hemiplegia.

(2) It strengthens the legs.

10. EKAPADAPRASARANASANA

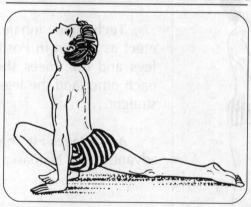

Ekapadaprasaranasana

Technique : Raise the trunk so that it is perpendicular to the floor and bring the left leg forward. Rest it at its original position and stretch the right leg backwards with the heels completely on the floor. The stomach should be pressed well in this position. Bring the neck and the head back and look as far back as possible.

Advantages : Blood circulates rapidly in the legs. One who practises this asana increases his capacity to walk and achieves flexibility in the spine.

11. HASTAPADASANA

Technique : Assume the position as shown in Hastapadasana. Pull the stomach inwards. Bring the other leg to its original position. Let the nose or the forehead touch the knees. Exhale.

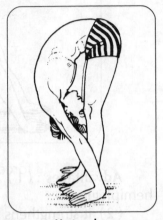

Hastapadasana

Advantages : It has all the advantages of Hastapadasana.

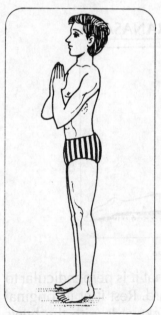

Namaskarasana

12. NAMASKARASANA

Technique : Inhale and stand erect as shown in Position 2. The legs and the knees should touch each other and the legs should be straight.

Advantages : It has all the advantages of Namaskarasana.

13. PRANAYAMA

The meaning of Pranayama : 'Pranayama' literally means 'to expand Prana' (vital force). In the 49th Sutra of Sadhanapada of Patanjala Yogasutra, the great Rishi Patanjali has defined Pranayama as a process in which respiration is interrupted and Prana, that is, the vital force is controlled and regulated. According to some, Prana means air. But this is a wrong and misleading interpretation. Prana means something more than air. Prana, in fact, is the vital power which is the force motivating every element of the earth and which is the origin of the force of thought. There is a deep affinity between Prana and mental force, between mental force and intellect, between intellect and soul, and between soul and God. Thus, the purpose of Pranayama is to inspire, motivate, regulate and balance the vital force (Prana) pervading in the body. This is the reason why Pranayama is considered one of the efficacious means of attaining Yoga.

The importance of Pranayama : Much importance has been attached to Pranayama in Yogashastras. According to Vyasabhashya, there is no 'tapa' (penance), greater than Pranayama. It cleanses the body and knowledge is manifested. Manu says, 'Just as gold and other metals melted in fire become pure so also the sense organs of the body get rid of impurities by Pranayama.' Pranayama is the fourth and very important stage of Ashtanga Yoga shown by Patanjali. Yoga without Pranayama is not Yoga at all. That is why Pranayama is called the soul of Yoga. Bathing is necessary for purifying the body. Similarly, Pranayama is essential for purifying the mind.

Advantages : (1) Pranayama keeps the body fit and healthy. It reduces excessive fat.

(2) One can live a long life through Pranayama. Pranayama improves the power of memory and eliminates mental disorders.

(3) Pranayama tones up the stomach, the liver, the bladder, the small and the large intestines and the digestive system.

(4) Pranayama purifies tubular channels and removes sluggishness from the body.

(5) Pranayama kindles gastric fire, the body becomes healthy and the inner voice begins to be heard.

(6) The constant practice of Pranayama strengthens the nervous system. The mind becomes calm and capable of concentration.

(7) The constant practice of Pranayama rouses spiritual power. It gives spiritual joy, spiritual light and mental peace.

Hints : For the effective and proper study of Pranayama, an aspirant should strictly follow the following hints :

(1) Pranayama should be practised in a clean, airy place. It should be practised in complete solitude.

(2) The best time for practice is the early morning. If this time is unsuitable, one may practise it in the evening.

(3) Pranayama is best done sitting on the floor. The postures suitable are Padmasana or Siddhasana. If one experiences difficulty in sitting in these postures for a longer time, one can select any convenient posture to sit steadily in an erect posture.

(4) The tubular channels should be cleansed before practising Pranayama. For this, first practise asanas.

(5) Pranayama should be performed at a chosen time regularly on an empty stomach. A small cup of milk, if taken at the interval of ten minutes, will serve as a good tonic.

(6) Do not practise Pranayama if you feel exhausted. The aspirant should feel fresh and active after the practice of Pranayama.

(7) Do not take bath immediately after the practice of Prahayama. Rest for half an hour before taking bath.

(8) According to Patanjali, one should inhale and exhale slowly and rhythmically during the practice of Pranayama. Rhythmic and slow breathing makes the mind steady and calm.

(9) A beginner of Pranayama should practise inhaling and exhaling only for a few days. The ratio of inhaling (puraka) and exhaling (rechaka) should respectively be 1 : 2. This means that the time spent in exhaling should be twice the time spent in inhaling.

(10) The time for retention of the breath (kumbhaka) should be increased gradually. In the first week, it should be for four seconds only; in the second, it should be for eight seconds and in the third, it should be for twelve seconds. In this way, one can gradually increase the time of retention of breath to one's utmost capacity.

(11) While inhaling, retaining the breath and exhaling, one must not experience any feeling of suffocation or strenuous effort.

(12) Maintain the ratio of 1 : 4 : 2 for inhaling, retention of breath and exhaling respectively. Inhale till you speak one Omkara. Retain the breath till you finish four Omkaras and exhale with two Omkaras. The following week the ratio should be 2 : 8 : 4, in the third week it should be 3 : 12 : 6 and so on. The limit is 16 : 64 : 32. Make the use of the fingers of the left hand for counting 'Om'. After some practice, counting becomes unnecessary. Habit will, of its own accord, maintain the proper ratio of puraka, kumbhaka and rechaka i.e., inhaling, retention of breath and exhaling.

(13) Do not get disturbed if a few mistakes are committed in the early stage. Do not give up the practice. How to maintain the ratio of puraka, kumbhaka and rechaka will be learnt automatically. Common sense, intuition and the spiritual voice will guide one to the path of accomplishment.

(14) Surya Bhedana and Ujjayi should be practised in winter only. Sitakari and Shitali should be practised in summer only. Bhastrika may be practised round the year.

Important guidelines regarding Pranayama : It is necessary for an aspirant to understand and grasp certain important items related to Pranayama. These important items are as follows :

(1) The technique of Pranayama

(2) Puraka (Inhaling), Kumbhaka (Retention of the breath) and Rechaka (Exhaling)

(3) Nadis–the Ida, the Pingala and the Sushumna

(4) Mula Bandha, Jalandhar Bandha and Uddiyana Bandha

(5) Nadishuddhi

(6) Kapalabhati

A brief explanation of these important aspects of Pranayama has been given below :

(1) The technique of Pranayama :
The left and right nostrils are to be closed for the practice of Pranayama. This is done mostly with the right hand. The right thumb is used to close the right nostril and the third and the fourth fingers are used to close the left nostril. When the holding of the nostrils is not required, keep the hands on the knees. For practising Pranayama, try to attain the posture of Padmasana, Siddhasana, Swastikasana and Sukhasana.

(2) Puraka, Kumbhaka and Rechaka
The meanings of these three important components of Pranayama are as are given below :
Puraka means to inhale.
Kumbhaka means to retain the breath.
Rechaka means to exhale.
Antarika Kumbhaka means retention following inhalation. Bahya Kumbhaka means restraint after exhalation. If Kumbhaka is taken with Rechaka and Puraka, it is known as 'Sahita Kumbhaka', if it is taken without Rechaka and Puraka, it is known as 'Kevala Kumbhaka'. One should practise Sahita Kumbhaka until Kevala Kumbhaka is accomplished.

(3) Ida, Pingala and Sushumna : Energy or lifeforce flows through these three Nadis (tubular channels). Their deities are the Moon, the Sun and the Fire respectively. The Ida starts from the left nostril, the Pingala from the right nostril and the Sushumna where both the nostrils meet. Hence the Sushumna is considered to be the 'central channel' (Madhya

Nadi). The Ida (left) and the Pingala (right) change their sound hourly.

The Ida is also called the nadi of the Moon. It is cool and has an element of 'Tamas'. It regulates human thoughts.

The Pingala is also called the nadi of the sun. It is warm and has an element of 'Rajas'. It regulates energy or lifeforce in human body.

The Sushumna is also called the Brahmanadi. Of all nadis, the Sushumna is the most important. In some books, it has been named as 'Saraswati' or 'Shanti' nadi. This nadi is neither warm nor cool but it is moderate. This nadi imparts wisdom and knowledge. It helps an aspirant in his spiritual progress.

From the physical point of view, the co-ordination of these three nadis gives health, strength, mental peace and long life.

(4) **Moola Bandha, Jalandhara Bandha and Uddiyana Bandha :** These three 'Bandhas' are chiefly performed during the practice of Pranayama. The techniques and the advantages of these three Bandhas have been given below :

MOOLA BANDHA

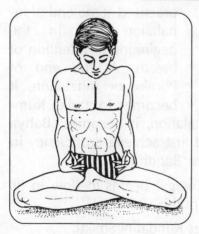

Moola Bandha

Technique : Press the lower abdominal muscle with the right heel and place the left heel at the root of the genitals. Contract the anal sphincter muscle upwards to the spine and feel the sensation that 'apana vayu' is drawn up. The exercise can be done replacing the left leg for the right one.

Advantages : (1) This 'Bandha' enables the aspirant to accomplish accuracy in Pranayama.

(2) The practice of this Bandha helps to maintain celibacy.

(3) It kindles gastric fire, eliminates constipation and nourishes virility.

(4) It awakens the Kundalini.

(5) The aspirant of this Bandha enjoys youth for a very long time.

JALANDHARA BANDHA

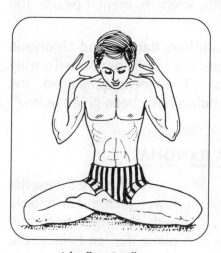

Jalandhara Bandha

Technique : Assume the sitting posture. Contract the neck and the throat (glottis) and bring the head low. Press the chin firmly against the chest.

Jalandhar Bandha is practised at the end of inhalation and in the beginning of retention of breath. At the end of Puraka or inhalation, it becomes 'Antarika Kumbhaka' and at the end of exhalation, it becomes 'Bahya Kumbhaka'. A beginner should first achieve proficiency in Pranayama before practising this 'Bandha'.

Advantages : (1) Prana (Energy) begins to flow in its proper channel by the practice of this 'Bandha'.

(2) This Bandha sublimates Kundalini Shakti.

(3) This Bandha closes the Ida and the Pingala 'nadis'.

UDDIYANA BANDHA

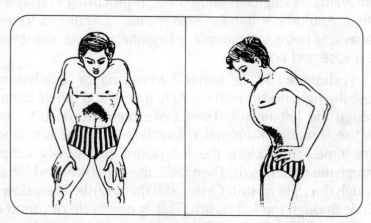

Uddiyana Bandha

Technique : This Bandha can be practised in either standing posture or sitting posture. In the standing posture, place the hands slightly above the knees. Bend the body slightly forward. Keep the legs apart. Exhale with full force. Now contract the abdomen and pull it upwards and backwards to the spine with the force of the navel and the diaphragm. The diaphragm will be pulled up and the abdominal wall will be pushed up to the back. This Bandha is practised after 'Kumbhaka' and before 'Rechaka'.

Advantages : (1) One who practises Uddiyana Bandha regularly attains eternal youth.

(2) This 'Bandha' helps in preserving celibacy.

(3) It awakens Kundalini Shakti.

(4) The constant practice of this Bandha makes the body vigorous and healthy.

Note : (1) All these three 'Bandhas' should be practised first with the help of either Siddhasana or Padmasana.

(2) When these three Bandhas are practised simultaneously, they are called 'Tribandha'.

(5) **Nadi Shuddhi or Anuloma-Viloma Pranayama :** Pranayama can be best performed after the purification of the tubular channels. Pranayama which is performed for the purification of tubular channels is called 'Anuloma-Viloma' Pranayama. A beginner should begin practising Pranayama with Anuloma-Viloma Pranayama. Anuloma-Viloma Pranayama being very simple, a beginner can practise it with great ease and comfort.

Technique : Sit in either Padmasana or Siddhasana. Close the right nostril with the right thumb and inhale deeply through the left nostril. Then close both the nostrils, and practise 'Antarika Kumbhaka' (holding air in the lungs) for some time. Then close the left nostril and slowly exhale through the right nostril. Then close the left nostril and inhale through the right nostril. Close both the nostrils. Then slowly exhale through the left nostril. This is one cycle or round of Nadi Shuddhi Pranayama. Practise three or four rounds every day and gradually increase the number of rounds. When you master this practice, follow the set rhythm in ratio of 1 : 2 : 2 for this exercise which means four seconds for inhalation, eight seconds for retention of breath and eight seconds for exhalation. After a long practice, proceed to 1 : 4 : 2 which means if inhalation takes five seconds, retention of breath should be for twenty seconds and exhalation should take ten seconds.

Advantages : (1) This is considered to be the best variation of Pranayama. It cures the diseases of the lungs.

(2) It helps blood to get a large supply of oxygen with the result that blood is well purified.

Note : A person with abnormal blood pressure should not attempt Kumbhaka. They should practise Puraka and Rechaka only. They should gradually begin practising Kumbhaka only after their blood pressure is normal.

(6) **Kapalabhati :** In Sanskrit, Kapala means 'skull' and 'Bhati' means 'to shine'. Thus, Kapalabhati is an exercise the practice of which imparts glow to the skull. It is one of the six purification exercises known to Hatha Yoga. Kapalabhati qualifies as aspirant for Bhastrika Pranayama.

Technique : Sit in either the Padmasana or the Siddhasana position. Place the hands on the knees. Lower the eyes. Inhale and exhale quickly and forcefully like the bellows of a blacksmith. This exercise should be done with full force so that the body perspires.

In Kapalabhati, Kumbhaka is not practised. Rechaka plays a significant part in this exercise. This is a very potent exercise. During the practice of Kapalabhati, the cells, the nerves and the muscles get a violent tremor.

Start with one exhalation in a second. Then gradually increase the speed to get two exhalations in a second. In the beginning, complete one cycle of ten exhalations. Then gradually increase the cycles.

Advantages : (1) Kapalabhati clears the skull, the respiratory system and the nasal cavities.

(2) As Kapalabhati eliminates the cough accumulated in the wind-pipe, asthma is cured.

(3) This exercise supplies plenty of oxygen to the air-cases (*alveoli*) in the lungs preventing viruses like the tuberculous bacilli from doing any damage to them.

(4) It draws out a large quantity of carbon dioxide from the body and thus purifies blood.

(5) It tones up the heart and activates the respiratory system, the circulatory system and the digestive system.

VARIETIES OF PRANAYAMA

Pranayama has many variations depending upon the type of Kumbhaka. According to Yogashastra, the following are the eight principal Kumbhakas :

(1) Surya Bhedana, (2) Ujjayi, (3) Sitakari, (4) Shitali, (5) Bhastrika, (6) Bhramari, (7) Moorchchha and (8) Plavini.

Each of the eight varieties of Pranayama has been described below with its technique and advantages so that an aspirant can make the best study of it.

1. Surya Bhedana

'Surya Bhedana' means piercing the Pingala nadi. The chief object of Pranayama is to rouse the Pingala nadi. The

Surya Bhedana exercise stimulates that part of the brain which contains Purusha Shakti i.e., the lifeforce (vital force). The practice of Surya Bhedana produces heat in the body. Therefore, this exercise is more beneficial during winter.

Technique : Sit in the Padmasana or the Siddhasana position. Close the eyes. Close the left nostril with the little finger of the right hand. Inhale deeply through the right nostril. Then close the right nostril with the right thumb. Rest the chin in the notch between the collar bone just above the breast bone. (This is Jalandhara Bandha.) Now practise Kumbhaka (Retention of breath). Gradually, increase the time for Kumbhaka. Then close the right nostril with the thumb and exhale slowly through the left nostril. Repeat this exercise in the same order.

Advantages : (1) The constant practice of this Pranayama purifies the mind and cures intestinal diseases.

(2) This Pranayama cures rheumatism and the diseases related to 'vata' (windiness). Moreover, it is the best remedy for blood impurities, skin diseases and leucoderma.

(3) It rouses 'Kundalini Shakti' which kindles gastric fire.

(4) It invigorates the liver and bile is produced in a sufficient quantity.

Note : Unhealthy persons should practise this Pranayama in winter and in monsoon sitting under the light rays of the rising sun or in the moderate rays of the setting sun in the evening.

2. Ujjayi

Heat is created in the body with the practice of 'Ujjayi' Pranayama. So it is advisable to practise it in winter.

Technique : Sit in the position of Padmasana or Siddhasana. Close the mouth. Contract the lower part of the tongue and the glottis and inhale rapidly and deeply through both the nostrils and fill the lungs up to the brim. Then practise

Kumbhaka for as much time as possible. Then close the right nostril with the right thumb and slowly exhale through the left nostril. While inhaling, expand the thoracic cage. This makes a faint sobbing sound as the glottis is half-closed.

Advantages : (1) This Pranayama reduces the heat of the head and cures asthma, tuberculosis and other diseases of the lungs.

(2) It kindles the gastric fire and activates the digestive system, the respiratory system and the nervous system.

3. Sitakari

The practice of Sitakari has a cooling effect on the body and hence it is beneficial to practise it in summer. Sitakari Pranayama immediately quenches thirst.

Technique : Sit in the position of Padmasana or Siddhasana. Let the tip of the tongue touch the palate. The middle part of the tongue should touch the lips. Draw the air in through the mouth with a sibilant sound (si ... si ... si ...). Hold the breath for as much time as possible. Then exhale through the nostrils.

Advantages : (1) Sitakari Pranayama relieves one of hunger, thirst, sluggishness and drowsiness.

(2) It eliminates harshness of the gland known as Rudragranthi.

(3) This Pranayama prevents bile from increasing.

(4) The constant practice of this Pranayama increases the physical strength and elevates the mental power of the aspirant.

4. Shitali

This Pranayama is very much beneficial in the spring and in summer seasons. This Pranayama cools the body and the mind. There is not much difference between Sitakari Pranayama and Shitali Pranayama. One should practise this Pranayama for fifteen to twenty minutes daily in the morning.

Technique : Sit in the position of Padmasana, Siddh-asana or Vajrasana. Protrude the tongue out and curl it like a pipe. Breathe with a sibilant sound (si... si... si) to fill the lungs completely. Hold the breath for as much time as possible. Then slowly exhale through both the nostrils.

Advantages : (1) This Pranayama purifies blood reliev-ing the body of toxic elements accumulated in it.

(2) This Pranayama cures diseases like tumour, enlargement of the spleen, skin diseases, fever, indigestion and constipation.

(3) This Pranayama quenches (relieves) thirst.

(4) The poison of a scorpion or snake has no effect on a regular practitioner of this Pranayama.

(5) This Pranayama is beneficial to persons having hot temperament.

(6) This Pranayama prevents flatulence, splenomegaly, excess of bile and cures leprosy.

5. Bhastrika

In Sanskrit, Bhastrika means 'bellows'. This exercise is characterized by continual exhalation of breath, producing a sound similar to a blacksmith's bellows. It is a combination of Kapalabhati and Ujjayi, Bhastrika is the most beneficial of all the Kumbhakas.

Technique : Sit in the position of Padmasana or Siddh-asana. Keep the body, the neck and the head erect. Place the hands on the knees or on the laps. Close the mouth. Breath fast and vigorously and exhale fast and forcefully like bellows. Repeat this in quick successive jerks five to ten times. Similarly, contract and expand the lungs. While practising this Pranayama, there will be a sound resembling air rushing through the bellows. An aspirant should inhale and exhale continually and quickly. When one cycle of inhalation and exhalation is completed, the aspirant should take a deep breath and hold it for as much time as possible without reaching the point of exhaustion. Then exhale. This is one cycle of

Bhastrika. Then breath in a normal way for some time and rest for a while. This will give some relief and prepare the aspirant for fresh cycles of Bhastrika. Practise three such cycles every morning, and if possible, practise two or three cycles in the evening. Busy persons, if unable to practise three cycles, should practise one cycle only. Even one cycle is enough for perfect health.

In winter, Bhastrika may be practised in the morning and in the evening, but in summer it should be practised only in the coolness of the morning.

Advantages : (1) Bhastrika reduces the swelling in the throat. It kindles gastric fire and removes cough. It cures chest-ailments, asthma and tuberculosis.

(2) Bhastrika cures all the diseases caused by phlegm, windiness and bile (Kafa, Vata and Pitta).

(3) Bhastrika unlocks the mouth of the Sushumna nadi.

(4) It gives temporary warmth to the body.

6. Bhramari

The word Bhramari is derived from Bhramara which means a black bee. While practising this Pranayama, the sound produced through the nostrils resembles the buzzing of a black bee.

Technique : Sit in the position of Padmasana or Siddhasana. Inhale and exhale quickly through the nostrils. Practise this till the body perspires. Then inhale deeply through the nostrils and hold the breath for as much time as possible. Then exhale through the nostrils. In the beginning, quick breathing stimulates blood circulation and heat of the body increases, but, in the end it is cooled down on account of perspiration and the joy experienced at this juncture is indescribable.

Advantages : (1) The practice of Bhramari delights the mind. One begins to acquire knowledge and emancipation from passion and worldly pleasures.

(2) One who gets success in practising Kumbhaka through Bhramari successfully enters the stage of Samadhi.

Note : Fresh aspirants will not derive much benefit out of this Pranayama unless they practise Anuloma-Viloma Pranayama.

7. Moorchchha

An aspirant practising this Pranayama falls into a swoon and he remains in an unconscious state. Hence this Pranayama is called 'Moorchchha'.

Technique : Sit in any comfortable position. Inhale through both the nostrils. Then practise deep Jalandhar Bandha and hold the breath. Then exhale through the nostrils.

Advantages : (1) As the mind remains in an unconscious state, the aspirant experiences spiritual joy.

(2) This Pranayama brings the mind in the profound state of quietude. According to Yogashastra, 'mana' (the mind) becomes amana that is non-existent. In other words, it is in communion with the Supreme Power.

8. Plavini

Plavini means that which makes one swim. Plavini Pranayama enables an aspirant to swim in water. Some skill is required for practising this Pranayama. The prolonged practice of this Pranayama enables the aspirant to swim in deep water for a long time. His body swims on the surface of the water like a lotus leaf.

Technique : In the beginning, this Pranayama should be practised sitting in the position of Siddhasana or Vajrasana. Then one can practise it in a standing or lying position. After assuming the sitting posture, inhale through the nostrils and hold the breath. Practise Jalandhar Bandha. Jalandhar Bandha causes breath to fill the intestines and this expands them profusively. At the completion of this Pranayama, exhale through both the nostrils. If necessary, exhalation can be done through belching or Uddiyana Bandha.

Advantages : (1) The aspirant of Plavini Pranayama can live upon only air for several days without taking food. (2) This Pranayama stimulates blood circulation. Consequently, all the toxic elements or impurities in the body are expelled.

Note : This Pranayama needs slow, gradual and regular practice. It should be practised under the proper guidance of one, who is proficient in Pranayama.

14. YOGASANA AND PRANAYAMA

Yogasana and Pranayama are closely inter-related. An aspirant should master asanas like Padmasana, Siddhasana, Swastikasana and Sukhasana before he begins to practise Pranayama. One can be called the master of a particular asana only when one practises it for three hours without any movement of the body. At the start, it is very difficult to accomplish this. So it is advisable to begin with any asana suitable to oneself him and practise Anuloma-Viloma Pranayama. Gradually, with the help of Pranayama, one will get mastery over that asana. Thus, Pranayama is helpful in getting mastery over asanas.

Yogasanas become much more effective if they are performed with Puraka, Kumbhaka and Rechaka Pranayama in the right proportion. Pranayama is helpful in practising and maintaining asanas. The lungs can be properly expanded and contracted through Yogasanas and Pranayama. Yogasanas and Pranayama supply plenty of oxygen to the lungs and so the body becomes healthy and the mind contented and delightful. Hence, the basic knowledge of Pranayama is of immense help to the students of Yogasana.

---

15. YOGASANA AND EXERCISES FOR THE CARE OF THE EYES

Of all the sense organs, the eye is most vital. Without sight, the world is nothing.

The science of Yoga has definitely recommended 'Tratak' to strengthen the sight. But if 'tratak' is not practised properly, it may damage the eyes.

Simhasana is one of the asanas which are beneficial to sight and the eyes. How to practise it is fully explained on page No. 35. Besides this asana, the asanas such as 'Sheershasana' and 'Sarvangasana' are indirectly beneficial to the eyes. Other exercises which are beneficial to sight and which strengthen and activate the eyes are given below :

(1) Eye-pressing :

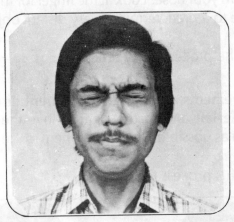

Press the eyes with the help of the muscles around the eyes and the muscles of the lids. Maintain this pressure for a few seconds (5–10 seconds). Then relax the muscles and the eyes as much as possible.

Repeat this exercise ten times.

(2) Alternately looking at near and distant objects :

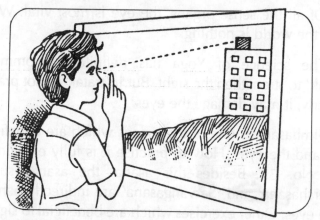

Stand near the window or in the balcony of the house. Hold the first (index) finger of the right hand about an inch or two away from your nose. Look at the finger for three seconds. Shift the gaze to a predetermined very distant object for three seconds.

Repeat the process thirty times.

(3) Movements of the eyes to different directions :

1. To the left and to the right : Move the eyes to the right as much as possible. Then move them to the left as much as possible.

Repeat this process ten times.

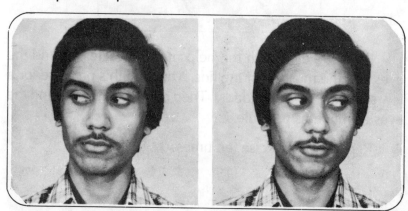

2. Upward and downward : Move the eyes upward as much as possible. Then bring them downwards as much as possible.

Repeat this process ten times.

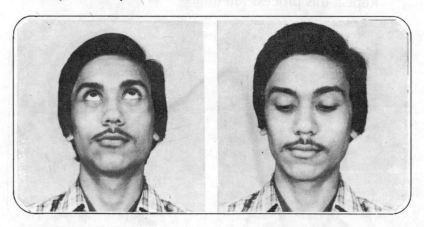

3. Upward to the left : Move the eyes to the corner of the left side. Then move them to the lower corner of the right side.

Repeat this process ten times.

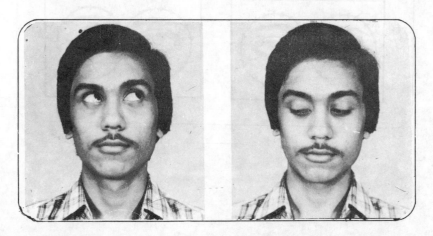

4. To the right side : Move the eyes to the upper corner of the right side. Then move them to the lower corner of the left side.

Repeat this process ten times.

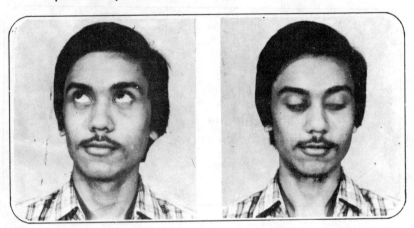

5. Circular movement : Move the eyes first in the clockwise direction and then in the anticlockwise direction. Continue each circular movement ten times.

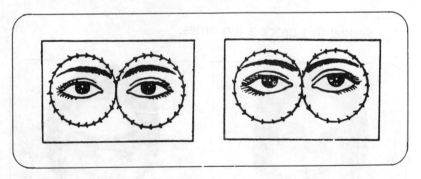

16. A SUITABLE DIET

The reader may ask why there should be a discussion on diet in this book of yoga.

In fact, one who desires to make progress in yoga, should seriously ponder over one's own diet. An improper diet is an obstacle to the study of yoga. One who does not care for one's diet does not get expected benefits through yoga.

A proper diet not only nourishes the body but also works as nectar, while an improper diet works as poison and damages the body in various ways. As a matter of fact, a diet affects not only health but also nature. There is a proverb, 'As is the tree so is the fruit'. In the same manner, we may say, **'As is the diet so is the health'.** It is commonly known that vegetarians are of peaceful nature, while non-vegetarians are of hot nature.

The diet of the persons practising yoga : Whatever we eat can generally be considered as diet. It consists of concrete things such as solid food, drinks, air and light and abstract things such as thoughts, imagination and feelings. In all the ancient books of yogashastra, suitableness and unsuitableness of a particular diet (food-commodity) has been explained. Hathayoga Pradeepika says, 'one's diet should be nutritious, sweet, oily and it should nourish virility. Moreover, it should please and satisfy the mind and should be agreeable to the taste.'

पुष्टं सुमधुरं स्निग्धं धातुप्रपोषणम्।
मनोभिलषित योग्यं योगी भोजनमाचरेत्॥

This kind of food is called sattvika.

Ancient books advise that the food which is excessively bitter, sour, saltish, pungent, hot or cold should not be given place in the diet. They also advise that one should avoid liquor, intoxicating things, fish, meat, eggs, asafoetida, garlic, onions and such other lustful (rajasika) food items in one's diet.

Furthermore, according to yogashastra, stale, tasteless, rotten or stinking food item should be avoided.

In other words, the ancient books on yoga tell us that such food as would obstruct and destroy physical, mental and emotional balance and equanimity should not be taken. Rajasika (lustful) and tamasika (vicious) food produces undesirable effects on the body and the mind. Yoga is a path to control the body and the mind and so it is natural that rajasika or tamasika food items have no place in the diet of those who practise yoga.

Yogashastra gives much importance to the goodness (Sattvikata) of food. Sattvika food consists of fruits, vegetables, cereals, milk, curd, buttermilk, butter and ghee. These food items supply all the necessary constituents required by the body. For example, fruits and vegetables provide precious vitamins and minerals to the body. These constituents enable the body to resist diseases. Furthermore, fruits and vegetables contain fibres which prevent or cure constipation. It is a common experience that one who suffers from constipation cannot practise asanas well. Cereals provide mostly carbohydrates to the body. These constituents give heat to the body. Butter and ghee provide fat to the body. This constituent also provides the body with heat. Besides, it oils the joints. Proteins are available from milk, curd and buttermilk. This constituent is necessary for the constitution of the body and the reconstruction of the cells.

The yogashastra describes 'how much to eat' together with 'what to eat'. That yogashastra lays emphasis on 'mitahar' (temperance in eating). Several yogashastras have suggested that while eating one should fill half the stomach with food, a quarter of stomach with water and the remaining quarter for free movement of air.

अन्नेन पूरयेदर्धं तोयेन तु तृतीयकम् ।

उदरस्य तृतीयांशं संरक्षेत् वायुचारणे ।। – धेरंडसंहिता

द्वौ भागौ पूरयेदनैस्तोयेनैकं प्रपूरयेत् ।

वायो: संचरणार्थाय चतुर्थमवशेषयेत् ।। – हठयोग प्रदीपिका

Owing to modern materialism, man has become the

victim of a badly adjusted diet. We do not eat to live but live to eat. Our diet has growingly become soft and spicy. We eat this type of food excessively. Very often we are misled by advertisements which say 'Eat as much as you want and digest it with our medicines'. Excessive eating is a burden to the digestive organs. The result is that we suffer from indigestion and gas. It also causes obesity.

Indigestion, gas and obesity are the three factors which obstruct the practice of asanas and hinder the path to 'Sadhana'.

In short, those who practise yoga should take simple and nourishing food in less quantity. If this rule is not observed, it is difficult to get mastery over asanas (the body) and impossible to get control over mana (the mind).

17. MODEL YOGASANA–TIMINGS

Here, three courses of study have been presented in order for inexperienced, moderately experienced and experienced persons practising yoga. Changes in them may be made in accordance with individual requirements and the convenience of time.

1. INITIAL YOGASANA–TIMINGS

1. Vajrasana 1 to 3 minutes 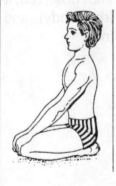	2. Ardha Pavanmuktasana 10 to 30 seconds; 2 to 4 times 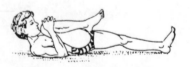
3. Ekapada Uttanasana 10 seconds; 4 to 6 times 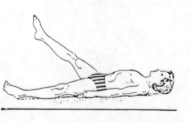	4. Supta Bhadrasana 10 to 30 seconds; 2 to 4 times 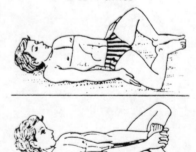

5. Bhujangasana
10 to 30 seconds;
4 to 6 times

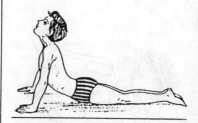

6. Ardha Shalabhasana
10 to 30 seconds;
5 to 7 times

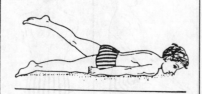

7. Padahastasana
2 to 10 seconds;
4 to 5 times

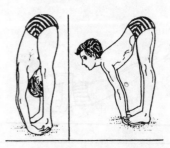

8. Trikonasana (2)
2 to 3 seconds;
4 to 5 times

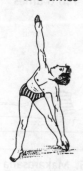

9. Shavasana
Convenient time;
5 to 10 minutes

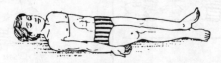

2. MADHYAM (MEDIUM) YOGASANA – TIMINGS

1. Vajrasana 1 to 3 minutes	2. Purna Pavanmuktasana 30 seconds; 2 to 4 times
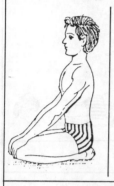 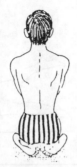	
3. Bhujangasana 30 seconds; 4 to 6 times	4. Purna Shalabhasana 30 seconds; 5 to 7 times
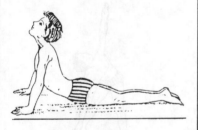	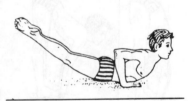
5. Makarasana 3 to 5 minutes	6. Utthita Dwipadasana 10 seconds; 4 to 6 times
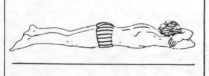	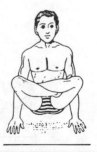

7. Pada Hastasana
10 to 15 seconds;
4 to 6 times

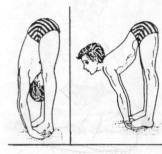

8. Trikonasana (2)
4 to 6 seconds;
4 to 6 times

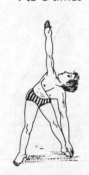

9. Janu Shirasana
8 to 10 seconds;
4 to 6 times

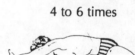
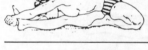
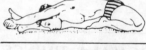
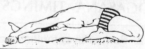

10. Vakrasana
30 seconds;
4 to 6 times

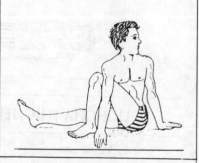

11. Halasana
10 to 30 seconds

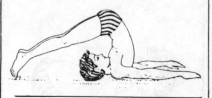

12. Bhoo-Namana-Vajrasana
10 to 30 seconds

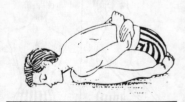

13. Viparitakarani Mudra
1 to 3 minutes

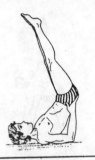

14. Pranayama (any kind)
1 to 3 minutes

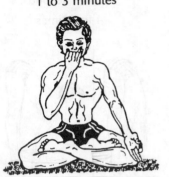

15. Shavasana
Convenient time;
5 to 10 minutes

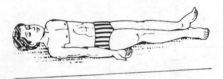

3. UCHCHA (HIGHER) YOGASANA–TIMINGS

1. Vajrasana
1 to 3 minutes

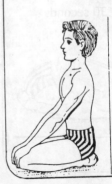

2. Purna Pavanmuktasana
30 seconds;
2 to 4 times

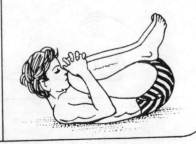

3. Bhujangasana
30 seconds;
4 to 6 times

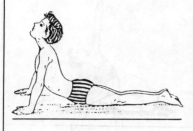

4. Purna Shalabhasana
30 seconds;
5 to 7 times

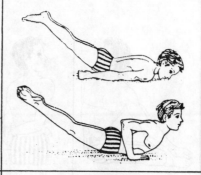

5. Dhanurasana
10 to 30 seconds;
4 to 6 times

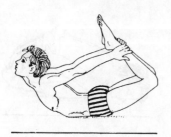

6. Makarasana
3 to 5 minutes

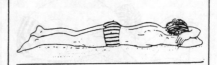

7. Tolangulasana
30 seconds;
4 to 6 times

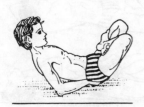

8. Halasana
30 seconds

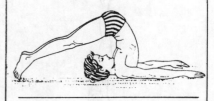

9. Purna Matsyendrasana
$\frac{1}{2}$ to 3 minutes

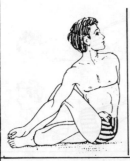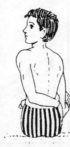

10. Trikonasana (2)
4 to 6 seconds;
4 to 6 times

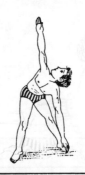

11. Pashchimottanasana
$\frac{1}{2}$ to 3 minutes

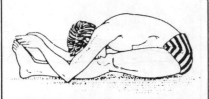

12. Bhoo-Namana-Vajrasana
30 seconds

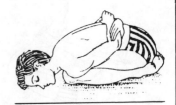

13. Sarvangasana
$\frac{1}{2}$ to 1 minute

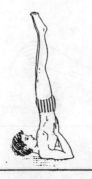

14. Matsyasana
10 to 30 seconds

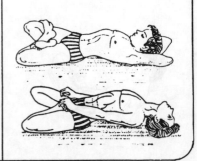

15. Parvatasana **10 to 30 seconds** 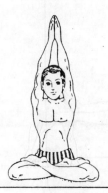	**16. Sheershasana** **30 to 60 seconds** 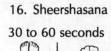 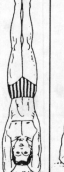 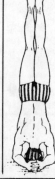
17. Shavasana **2 to 5 minutes** 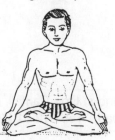	**18. Uddiyana Bandha** **According to** **one's capacity** 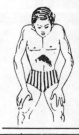 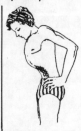
19. Kapalabhati One repetition with one exhaling. Increase the number gradually.	**20. Ujjayi** According to one's capacity 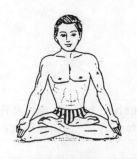

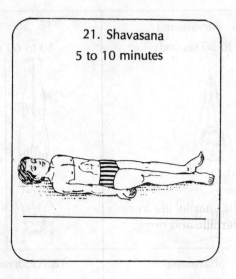

21. Shavasana
5 to 10 minutes

Published by   Navneet Publications (India) Ltd., Dantali, Gujarat.
Printed by   Dila Printers, Ahmedabad.   Tel. 212 01 23

FROM FAT TO FIT

**By reading this book you have
nothing to lose-expect your ugly fat.**

Do you believe that obesity only makes a person look ugly?
No. .... It also.

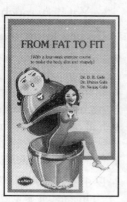

- robs a person of his opportunities of getting a good job or a suitable match.
- enhances the chances of developing many grave diseases.
- raises the rate of mortality due to liver problems.
- throws the marital life in disorder.
- reduces fertility and prevents conception.
- enhances the chances of developing diabetes, high blood-pressure and heart-disease.
- increases chances of developing cancer.
- shortens the life-span.

Reducing extra fat is essential not only for improving your figure and appearance, but also for good health. This book shows you sure and scientific ways to reduce extra fat.

Salient features of this Book :

- Interesting scientific information.
- A detailed-analysis of causes responsible for the development of obesity.
- A daily diet-plan for slimming.
- Exercises (with illustrations) to make the body healthy and proportionate.
- Practical suggestions at every step.

This book will not only teach you how to reduce your weight, but will also show you how to maintain your proper weight!

> **If you possess this book, there is no need
> for you to buy any other book on 'obesity'.**

PREVENT HEART DISEASE AND PROLONG LIFE

Heart is the most vital organ of our body.

Instant death would be a certainty if it stopped beating even for a short while.

Yet how much do you know about your heart?

Do you know that –

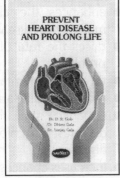

- the incidence of heart disease is rising at an alarming pace?
- of the total deaths in our country, 33% deaths occur due to heart disease?
- half of the total number of heart-patients pass away even before they reach a hospital?
- ignorance sows the seeds of heart disease in a person's life from his young age?

In fact, it is too late when a heart-attack strikes a person. Muscles and tissues of the heart are of a special type. Re-generation of those muscles and tissues is impossible once they are rendered dead by a heart-attack. And therefore, prevention of heart disease is the only alternative left to save the heart. Heart disease can be prevented by taking timely measures.

This book supplies you all the necessary, detailed and authentic information about all those measures.

Other unique features of this book :

- Interesting and scientific information, with illustrations, about the heart and heart disease.
- A thorough analysis of the factors and causes responsible for a heart-attack.
- A discussion on the symptoms and the treatment of a heart-attack.
- Detailed information regarding the steps that a layman would be required to take in an emergency when somebody's heart stops beating all of a sudden. If you follow those steps well, you can save someone's life and give him a fresh lease of life.
- A comparative study of the merits and demerits of coronary bypass surgery and transluminal coronary angioplasty.

A unique and unavoidable book for every individual who feels concerned for his own health and that of his dear ones.